T0398387

THE BURNOUT SOLUTION

The Burnout Solution

7 STEPS FROM
Exhausted to Extraordinary

Sharon Grossman, PhD

JOHNS HOPKINS UNIVERSITY PRESS
Baltimore

Johns Hopkins University Press
2715 North Charles Street
Baltimore, Maryland 21218
www.press.jhu.edu

Library of Congress Cataloging-in-Publication Data

Names: Grossman, Sharon, 1977– author.
Title: The burnout solution : 7 steps from exhausted to extraordinary /
    Sharon Grossman, PhD.
Description: Baltimore : Johns Hopkins University Press, 2025. |
    Includes index.
Identifiers: LCCN 2024048459 (print) | LCCN 2024048460 (ebook) |
    ISBN 9781421451985 (hardcover) | ISBN 9781421451992 (paperback) |
    ISBN 9781421452005 (ebook)
Subjects: LCSH: Burn out (Psychology)
Classification: LCC BF481 .G76 2025 (print) | LCC BF481 (ebook) |
    DDC 158.7/23—dc23/eng/20241231
LC record available at https://lccn.loc.gov/2024048459
LC ebook record available at https://lccn.loc.gov/2024048460

A catalog record for this book is available from the British Library.

*Special discounts are available for bulk purchases of this book. For more
information, please contact Special Sales at specialsales@jh.edu.*

EU GPSR Authorized Representative
LOGOS EUROPE, 9 rue Nicolas Poussin, 17000, La Rochelle, France
E-mail: Contact@logoseurope.eu

To Ariella and Ben:
May you find your calling,
be immersed in work
that inspires and challenges you,
and create a life filled with
vigor and joy.

Contents

A Note from the Author

Over the course of my career and through all of my personal development training, I learned some amazing tools, strategies, and mindsets for success. For a long time, I was on the receiving end of the information, consuming it like a thirsty soul. Eventually, however, I wanted to bring these powerful resources together in a meaningful way to benefit others.

Writing this book has been a gift through which I was able to put down on paper the essence of what has had impact on my life and that of my clients, and share it with the world.

During the process of writing, I noticed myself going through the seven steps.

- *Emotional intelligence*: It was the awareness of my strengths and my desire to write that catapulted this project.

- *Empowerment*: Over the two and a half years it took me to write this book, I often had to prioritize writing over other aspects of my business. I learned to minimize distractions and energy drains.

- *Engagement*: I became aware of how immersed I was in the writing. Hours would fly by, and when I would stop ever so briefly to check the time, I realized that I had forgotten to eat my lunch.

- *Efficacy*: Although it has been the longest process I've ever committed myself to (even longer than my doctoral dissertation), my belief in my ability to finish the project never wavered. I started out by writing long weekly entries for my blog and then stitched them together to create this book.

- *Energy*: I practice what I preach, and self-care has been an essential part of my journey that has helped move this book along. With few exceptions, I stuck to my wellness routines and paid close attention to my energy levels.

- *Effort*: Looking back at all the work I've poured into this book can give the impression that it took tremendous effort—and it did, but it did not feel overwhelming. I employed the idea of working smartly and making the most of my time.

- *Enlightenment*: Finally, I have reached the conclusion of this writing with a spring in my step, knowing that I have accomplished what I set out to do with the hope of enlightening those of you who need this book the most. From my heart to yours.

If it's your dream to thrive in your work and personal life, but burnout is getting you down, then set up a time to speak with me at www.drsharongrossman.com.

Remember to claim all the bonus materials from this book, which you can access at www.BurnoutToResilience.com:

- the accompanying workbook with all the book's exercises

- an infographic depicting the various ways burnout can manifest itself

- a guided breathing exercise to help you de-stress

- a gratitude template

- a guided loving-kindness meditation

- a grounding exercise called "Taking Down the Flame"
- a boundary-setting exercise to preserve and protect your energy
- a mindfulness meditation

THE BURNOUT SOLUTION

Introduction

WHY THIS BOOK MATTERS

Many of us dream of finding fulfillment in our careers. Yet the reality often falls short. This can stem from a lack of control over your work environment or internal struggles that prevent satisfaction. Burnout frequently emerges from this gap between expectation and reality.

The COVID-19 pandemic dramatically reshaped the way we work. Remote work, once a fringe concept, became the norm for millions. While this shift offered flexibility and work-life balance for many, it also presented new challenges, including increased isolation, blurred work-life boundaries, and the ever-present threat of burnout.

Excessive and prolonged stress at work, whether in the office or remote, can leave you emotionally, physically, and mentally drained. Burnout is that feeling of being overwhelmed and underappreciated. It takes a toll and leads to a decline in motivation and performance.

What's particularly frustrating is that burnout can mimic other mental health conditions, such as depression and anxiety. You might experience persistent sadness, lose interest in work, feel constantly fatigued or irritable, even develop nervousness—all of which can be symptoms of major depressive disorder or generalized anxiety disorder. But here's the key difference: Burnout stems primarily from chronic workplace stress and involves feelings of inefficacy, cynicism, and a diminished sense of professional ability. It's not about a general lack of interest in life, but a specific disillusionment with your work environment.

The World Health Organization (WHO) now recognizes burnout and includes it in their International Classification of Diseases. However, it's not classified as a medical condition. Instead, it's categorized as an occupational phenomenon, meaning it arises from work-related stress. This is where understanding burnout, its triggers, and its symptoms becomes crucial.

Even though I am obsessed with living a balanced life, I wasn't totally immune to burnout. Early in my career, I transitioned from nonprofit work to private practice. I had heard so much about other psychologists who had gone into private practice and burned out. That put me on a mission: I was going to do it smarter.

To ensure I would not burn out, I created a schedule that included breaks, healthy lunches, and midday exercise. I kept my office hours reasonable, not working early mornings, nights, or weekends. My excitement about having a successful private practice kept me feeling positive about my career. For a while.

Over time, I noticed that even with my mission to do it smarter, I had fallen into the "grind." I ended up doing the bare minimum. I was having session after session with clients and stopped feeling very engaged. Although I was paying attention during the sessions and really cared about my clients, I had stopped going above and beyond.

I was brought to this place of relative burnout because I'd lost touch with my purpose. When I realized this, I sat down and asked myself, "Why am I doing this work?" I connected to what drove my passion for wanting to help people live better lives, and because I knew I had what it takes to help them achieve happiness in their work, I got reconnected to my "why."

With this renewed sense of purpose, I started to prepare for my sessions. I came up with resources and exercises to challenge my clients and help them move beyond their "stuck points" and conflicts. I gave them ideas about what they could do in between sessions in order to continue to grow and learn.

In addition to my personal experience, I was learning from my clients. What I found is that burnout happens for different reasons, and you have to find your way back from it based on what got you there in the first place. In other words, the road to recovery is personal.

Whitney's and Eddy's experiences exemplify this perfectly.

A physician and former client, Whitney describes her experience with burnout and her recovery in this way:

> Years of negative thinking had gotten me into a technically "good place" in life where I was miserable—a scary place of burnout, fatigue, demoralization, and finally depression, despite doing yoga and meditation and seeking help from friends, family, and other therapists. I was and continue to be (happily) shocked at the change in perspective that working with Dr. Sharon helped me to make, and by the impact that it has had on my life. Most significant is my awareness of negative thinking and how it's not helpful—so I am able to let it go. And a shift toward self-compassion and trusting my own wisdom, as opposed to second-guessing myself and the world constantly. This shift has had a dramatic impact on my moment-to-moment contentedness, which has made me a more present, happy, and effective mother, doctor, mentor, friend, colleague, and wife.

Eddy, a dedicated nurse, was on track to achieve his dream of buying a house and starting a family. He readily put in extra hours, fueled by his long-term goals, but then everything changed when a coworker's bullying behavior created a hostile work environment.

Anxiety flooded Eddy, manifesting as debilitating knee pain that required surgery. Returning to work, he found himself consumed by worry, his energy and motivation plummeting. Sleep became elusive, replaced by constant rumination on his problems. Exhausted and unable to focus, Eddy became self-critical and irritable, a stark contrast to his usual self.

Through coaching, Eddy embarked on a journey of self-discovery. He worked on building his self-worth and letting go of the need for control. He reestablished self-care routines, practiced calming techniques to manage his anxiety, and rediscovered the joy of fun activities. Most importantly, Eddy challenged his belief that self-worth hinged on productivity. He learned to value himself as a person, not just his output. This shift allowed him to practice self-compassion and prioritize his own needs, and that transformed more than just his work life. He reclaimed his energy, confidence, and, above all, a healthy relationship with himself.

While my burnout stemmed from a loss of purpose, negative thinking was at the core of Whitney's burnout, and workplace bullying was what triggered Eddy's burnout. Each burnout story had a different starting point and different ways of manifesting, and each one required different solutions for recovery. This is what shaped my approach to burnout recovery not only in my coaching, but also in this book, throughout which you'll find a variety of mindsets, skill sets, and tool sets designed to address burnout's many faces. Don't feel pressured to use them all—pick and choose what resonates with you to create your unique path to recovery.

By sharing these lessons, I want to help you reignite the passion that drove you to your career. After all, you've likely invested years of education and training. This book, alongside my Exhausted to Extraordinary (E2E) Program, empowers you to leverage that investment, rediscover joy in your work, and finally reap the rewards of your dedication.

WHY YOU SHOULD READ THIS BOOK

Remember the game "M.A.S.H." from the 1980s? In this classic childhood game, players would write down names of potential spouses, locations to live, occupations, and number of children on separate slips of paper. By following a specific pattern of crossing out options, players would randomly determine their future. Back then, career aspirations were often about fame or fortune—doctor, lawyer, rock star. Fast forward to today, and the reality is quite different. Many high achievers in demanding fields such as medicine and law end up burned out, despite achieving success.

Burnout is a slow creep, not a sudden crash. You might not even recognize it in yourself until you hear the term, and the pieces click. That's why you need a framework, a roadmap to navigate the insidious symptoms and prevent burnout before it explodes. This book equips you with all the tools and components that make up the E2E framework.

The framework I speak of isn't a one-size-fits-all solution. It's the culmination of over 20 years of my experience as a psychologist and executive coach. Through countless client interactions,

I've iteratively honed this approach to tackle burnout from all angles, addressing stress management, emotional well-being, and productivity optimization. No matter where you are on the burnout spectrum, this framework offers support in three areas:

- *Early warning signs*: You'll learn to identify the subtle signs of burnout before they escalate.

- *Effective recovery strategies*: You'll discover practical tools to overcome burnout and reclaim your well-being.

- *Proactive prevention techniques*: You'll design a work-life balance that prevents burnout in the first place.

But this work isn't for everyone. As a coach, I look for clients who are WOW—worldly, open, and willing to do the work. The same applies for my consulting clients. If you are ready to ditch burnout and ignite passion in your team, the E2E framework is tailored for you.

WHAT YOU'LL LEARN IN THIS BOOK

This book isn't just a read—it's your personalized guide to overcoming burnout and building resilience. While the research and insights will inform you, the real power lies in taking action. Here's what's inside:

Part I: Understanding Burnout

We'll explore the stress-burnout continuum, so you can recognize warning signs and become stress-hardy. I explain all the ways burnout manifests so you can correctly diagnose it as it is happening and address it in its midst.

Part II: Active Practice

This section equips you with the first four steps of the E2E system to overcome burnout:

- *Emotional intelligence*: This involves developing your self-awareness, self-mastery, and relationship skills, which will equip you to navigate any situation effectively.

- *Empowerment*: Here, you'll identify where you gain and where you lose power. Distinguishing between the two can make a massive impact on your energy and overall well-being.

- *Engagement*: Next, you'll learn to engage in your work in a meaningful way by replacing disengagement with fulfillment and increased performance.

- *Efficacy*: This comes from building confidence in your abilities, which will allow you to take risks, learn, and grow.

Part III: Passive Presence

The final three steps focus on more passive techniques to maximize your efforts so you can be aligned with your purpose:

- *Energy management*: You'll explore strategies to protect and replenish your energy, the key to long-term productivity.

- *Effort optimization*: You'll learn to work smarter, not harder, by understanding the dynamics of motivation and effort.

- *Enlightenment*: You'll discover your core values and harness powerful tools to break through limitations and achieve lasting transformation.

How You Can Get the Most Out of This Journey

- *Bite-sized learning*: Each chapter is packed with clear information, followed by engaging exercises designed to be applied to your specific situation. Don't rush through—take your time to reflect and integrate the learnings before moving on. Think of me as your coach, guiding you step-by-step.

- *Active participation*: Ample space is provided within the book for your answers. However, consider keeping a dedicated notebook for in-depth journaling and tracking your progress throughout the entire program. This will serve as a powerful record of your transformation.

- *Digital toolkit*: Enhance your experience with the downloadable workbook available at www.Burnout ToResilience.com. This comprehensive resource includes printable versions of the exercises, along with bonus materials such as guided meditations to deepen your learning.

- *Tailored approach*: While there is a wealth of exercises and checklists, feel free to personalize your journey. Complete as many or as few as resonate with you. The key is taking action and actively participating in your own well-being.

The tools you'll find in this book are designed to create lasting change from the inside out, equipping you to thrive even in challenging situations. You'll learn to:

- reduce stress and work smarter, not harder
- boost your confidence and trust in your abilities

- quiet negativity and cultivate optimism
- create a life filled with balance, happiness, and ease.

Don't wait until burnout consumes you. Take control of your thoughts, feelings, and actions. Become the person who achieves their goals with energy to spare. This journey to reclaim your spark starts now. Turn the page, and let's begin.

FIGURE I.1   Your energy tank.

PART I

Understanding Burnout

CHAPTER 1

The Stress-Burnout Continuum

Stress arises when individuals perceive that they cannot adequately cope with the demands being made on them or with threats to their well-being.
RICHARD S. LAZARUS, *PSYCHOLOGICAL STRESS AND THE COPING PROCESS*

Stress is the arousal you experience when demands are placed on you if you perceive those demands to exceed your resources. Performance increases with stress to a point. The Human Function Curve (figure 1.1) depicts the point where this relationship peaks. As stress levels go up, you begin to experience tension. Once you pass your comfort zone, you reach the apex, named "The Hump."[1] This is the point where you have exceeded your resources and fatigue sets in. If stress continues to climb, causing exhaustion and poor health, productivity starts to decline. Ultimately, you will experience a breakdown. This breakdown is your burnout point.

Each of us has a different set point for where good stress turns into distress. According to research from the City University of New York, three characteristics define people who are stress-hardy.[2] The first characteristic correlates with how much *perceived* control a person thinks they have over a situation in front of them. To reduce the effects of a stressor, one needs to find ways to feel more in control. Faulty perceptions may cause you to see yourself as having less control than you do, so

FIGURE 1.1   The Human Function Curve. *Source*: Nixon, "The Human Function Curve."

changing such perceptions can positively affect your resilience, thus also improving your performance.

The second characteristic explains that stress-hardy individuals tend to be highly *committed* to and engaged in their tasks. By giving your work your full attention, you are changing the way you behave rather than having to change any external circumstances. Engagement, in turn, gives you more control over the situation so that you can focus on maximizing your returns.

The third characteristic has to do with the fact that when individuals are flexible in their thinking, they embrace change by seeing it as a *challenge* rather than a threat. Recognize that what worked for you in the past may not work now. It would be best if you found new ways to interact, adapt, and re-prioritize as change occurs.

TABLE 1.1 **Turn Your Stress Around**

1. Consider a work situation that currently feels highly stressful to you. In one sentence, write down what the situation is about.

   _____

   _____

2. Identify the root causes of stress, whether it's excessive workload, unrealistic deadlines, lack of support, or something else.

   _____

   _____

3. Pick one or more stress-hardy strategies (control, commitment, challenge) to turn your situation around.

   • How much control do you think you have in this instance? How did you come to that perception? If you could look at the situation from the perspective that you have more control, what would that look like?

   _____

   _____

   • How committed and engaged have you been in your tasks? Is something preventing you from being more fully committed? Identify what the obstacles are and then come up with a strategy to remove them and increase commitment.

   _____

   _____

   • If the stress you feel is due to a change you are facing, identify what thoughts are going through your mind about the change.

   _____

   _____

   Notice if you perceive the change as a threat. Then come up with a new way of thinking about the situation so that you see it instead as a challenge.

   _____

   _____

By shifting your perspective about what you have control over, how committed you are to your work, and what represents a challenge rather than a threat, you can increase your stress hardiness.

There are also three common ways people become overly stressed. Keep them in mind as you learn to avoid burnout.

Imagine that you are a frog jumping from rock to rock across a pond (figure 1.2). For this to be a reasonable challenge, each rock should be big enough for you to land on easily but not so big that you become stuck there. Similarly, your tasks at work should induce enough stress to motivate you, but not be overly taxing on your resources so that you experience an unhealthy degree of stress.

Now think of each rock as symbolizing a stressful episode. The number of jumps you have to take will affect your total energy level. Likewise, at work, you want to get through the day without too many stressful episodes.

Note, too, that before jumping to the next rock, you need time to recover your energy from the last jump. While it might be tempting to push yourself from one stressful episode to the next, you should instead take time to de-stress and regain your

FIGURE 1.2 Stress points on your journey.

energy before moving forward. Doing so will enable you to have the energy you need to complete your journey.

You might have incredibly high demands in any given task. Your job responsibilities might include too many stressful episodes that end up overwhelming you. Or, you might not have enough time to recover before moving on to the next challenge. Indeed, these circumstances can lead to burnout over time.

CONCLUSION

Stress can help or hinder your performance. To avoid burnout, you must pay attention to your energy levels and notice where fatigue sets in. Over time, when demands are incredibly high, when your job responsibilities are too many, or when you do not have enough time to recover between tasks, you can burn out. On the flip side, when you perceive yourself as having control, when you are committed to your work, and when you see it as challenging rather than threatening, you will become more stress-hardy.

CHAPTER 2

Identifying Burnout Triggers

In the same way that you and your neighbor might experience depression or happiness for different reasons, each of you can burn out for unique reasons. In this chapter we will uncover three main stressors that contribute to burnout: your work environment, your personality, and the interaction between the two.

ENVIRONMENTAL STRESSORS

When it comes to burnout stressors, it is easiest to start looking for the problems outside of yourself and then investigate personal contributing factors. To start, let's examine how your work environment can lead you to feel stressed. Consider three main work-related stressors: job demands, job resources, and control.

Job Demands

Job demands are defined as "aspects of the job that require sustained physical or mental effort and are therefore associated with certain physiological and psychological costs."[1] When you have too much on your plate, have sudden conflicts with co-workers, or prolonged worry about your job security, among many other things, you can become drained.

Demands can be emotional, mental, or physical, or they can arise from a work-home conflict. You might feel overwhelmed when there are excessive demands on your internal resources (e.g., time and energy), when the pace of change is too quick, when there are expectations of working long hours, or when deadlines become tighter. These high expectations can quickly deplete your energy reserves. Intense demands can also be non-verbal, as in work cultures where workers pride themselves on working overtime and not taking a lunch break. Adverse change, bureaucracy, harassment, and role or interpersonal conflicts are additional organizational factors that can feel taxing.

Prior to the COVID-19 pandemic, the trend among many Americans was to work long hours. A 2014 Gallup poll reported that nearly 40 percent of Americans worked over 50 hours per week, with almost 20 percent putting in over 60 hours.[2] However, the pandemic sparked a significant shift in workplace dynamics. Recent data from the Bureau of Labor Statistics shows that as of 2024, the average workweek for all employees on private nonfarm payrolls in the United States was 34.2 hours.[3] This shift reflects a growing emphasis on work–life balance and flexibility. Despite this overall trend, some sectors still see extended working hours. For instance, 94 percent of service professionals reportedly work over 50 hours per week.[4] However, research consistently shows that this heavy investment of time and energy does not pay off. A Stanford University study indicates that productivity steeply declines after 55 hours of work per week.[5] Moreover, a 2023 survey by Slack's Workplace Lab found that employees who log off at the end of the workday reported 20 percent higher productivity scores than those who feel pressured to work after hours.[6] All that results from that extra personal investment is often increased stress and diminished returns.

It is not just the demands of work that are eating people up. There is also life outside the office. There are people you care about, and to cultivate these relationships, whether they are friends, family members, a spouse, or children, you need time and energy after work. If your home life is also demanding, you are just not getting a break. You might soon realize this is not sustainable.

In an attempt to stay afloat on the work front, you might sacrifice your personal time. You stop going to the gym. You get home after the kids are already in bed. You have no time to unwind from work because you get home with barely enough time to eat, shower, and get to bed. You might even be taking work home. You keep coming back to the notion that "there's got to be a better way."

Job Resources

According to burnout researchers, there are various types of job resources whose purpose is to support the worker to achieve job-related goals, increase learning and personal growth, and reduce stress.[7]

Autonomy is one such resource. Self-Determination Theory states that autonomy is an innate psychological need that, when satisfied, allows the person to function more optimally. When we are given the freedom to act in harmony with our needs, we feel more in control, more respected, and more motivated.[8] When working autonomously under stress, we cope more adaptively because we feel like we have more choice in how and when to respond.

Social support is a resource that allows you to get more done in less time through high-quality relationships with colleagues and supervisors. It can include both instrumental support, such as help with technical difficulties or advice about how to deal with a difficult client, and emotional support, which helps you feel understood and validated.

Through constructive feedback, employees increase their work effectiveness. When you are recognized for good performance, your motivation soars. And when feedback focuses on problem areas, you can improve and overcome challenges more easily rather than remain stuck.

I often hear from my clients that their work lacks opportunities for growth. Once you have mastered the demands of your job, you seek to grow and be challenged anew. Autonomy can help you stay engaged and promote leadership and other critical skills that escalate your professional career.

Consider what resources your job provides that keep you motivated, engaged, and performing optimally. Then, consider what resources might be missing that, if you could access them, would make your job less stressful. The chapters in "Step 3: Engagement" provide a more in-depth look at additional types of job resources.

Demands and Resources

Stress does not result merely by being faced with excessive demands. There is more to it. Researchers Arnold Bakker and Evangelia Demerouti proposed a visual model that exemplifies how the combination of demands and resources affects employee well-being (figure 2.1).[9] Of the four possible combinations, three are unsustainable. Only one promotes wellness. This book looks in particular at the intersection of high job demands with low resources, which brings about burnout, and its polar opposite of high demands coupled with adequate resources which leads to work engagement.

As the model notes, the answer is not necessarily about lowering work demands. It is about looking at the interaction between demands and resources. When demands are low but resources are high, employees are prone to boredom. When demands and resources are both low, employees feel apathetic. Optimal performance results when demands and resources are in proper balance.

FIGURE 2.1   The Job Demands–Resources Model. *Source*: Bakker and Demerouti, "The Job Demands–Resources Model."

That said, we can further delve into how to distinguish between two different types of high demands.[10] Marcie Cavanaugh and colleagues looked at the amount of effort and energy tasks required and their respective outcomes. Together, these factors helped determine whether a demand is a challenge or a hindrance. *Challenge demands* are when you use your energy efficiently while investing effort into tasks and when these tasks result in learning, goal attainment, competence, or mastery. *Hindrance demands*, which can include interpersonal conflicts, require a considerable amount of effort and energy but lack positive outcomes related to growth. Thus, high demands can have different results depending on the rewards you get for your efforts.

Control

While job demands and resources play crucial roles in the development of burnout, the concept of control—or lack thereof—is another significant environmental factor that can contribute to workplace stress.

The relationship between control and workplace well-being is nuanced. As mentioned earlier, too little or too much control can wreak havoc on your experience at work. Lack of control is one of the main reasons for burnout, especially if the control you feel on the job does not match your desire for control.[11]

If you find yourself reporting to a boss who is a micromanager, you will likely want to have greater autonomy. We all aspire to have accountability and recognition for our efforts rather than have someone standing over us watching our every move. We feel micromanaging bosses don't trust us to get the job done right, similar to a parent who watches their kid like a hawk to make sure they do not hurt themselves or break something, always ready with a critique of how the child needs to be more careful.

Alternatively, Type A personalities, or those who are highly competitive and who have control, often do not delegate responsibility. Their work keeps piling up, but they want to do it all themselves, which leads to a sense of being overwhelmed.

Your relationship with control is not only based on your personality, but also related to where on the burnout spectrum you are. If you already feel worn out, making decisions will be difficult. To protect your energy, you will be more likely to avoid additional responsibilities.

There are many upsides to having control, including "more intrinsic motivation, greater interest, less pressure and tension, more creativity, more cognitive flexibility, better conceptual learning, a more positive emotional tone, higher self-esteem, more trust, greater persistence of behavior change, and better physical and psychological health."[12]

When we feel most out of control within, we focus on controlling the world without. Low control leads to lower levels of satisfaction and inner reward, which leads workers to demand more external rewards, including higher pay. And regardless of the truth of your situation, your perception of control is what matters. When you feel you have control, you feel less stressed and more capable of making good decisions.

Demands and Control

While demands and control are both stress-related factors, it is the interaction between them that can lead to burnout. This interaction is shown in the Job Demands–Control Model (figure 2.2).[13]

High-strain jobs are those in which demands are high and autonomy is low. While these types of jobs may suit a person who is motivated by challenges, it can still lead that person to work at a frenetic pace and subsequently feel exhausted.

Low-strain jobs, characterized by low demands and high autonomy, may seem ideal on paper. However, the lack of challenge inherent in these roles can lead to boredom and a sense of stagnation. Over time, this can contribute to decreased motivation and, ultimately, burnout. While autonomy can be empowering, it's essential to have a sufficient level of challenge to maintain engagement and job satisfaction.

Active jobs contain high demands and high autonomy. When you get to call the shots, you have less fear of change and are more likely to take risks. You just need to remain flexible in finding solutions to obstacles as they arise.

Passive jobs are ones where both demands and control are low. Under such circumstances, you are less likely to find pur-

FIGURE 2.2 The Job Demands–Control Model. *Source*: Karasek, "Job Demands, Job Decision Latitude, and Mental Strain."

pose or satisfaction in your work. This is usually the case in big bureaucracies that have workers follow an antiquated procedure. You do not feel strained by your work necessarily, but the lack of autonomy coupled with the lack of purpose may make work feel like just a way of getting your bills paid. The lack of challenge can, once again, lead to disengagement and boredom.

PERSONAL STRESSORS

The demands of a job itself are often what lead workers to the point of burnout.[14] While there is much truth to the fact that job sites are placing overwhelming demands on their workers while providing them with inadequate support, there is likely

TABLE 2.1 Balancing Demands with Resources

1. How many hours per week do you work on average?
   - ☐ Less than 40
   - ☐ 40–49
   - ☐ 50+

2. How do you manage the demands on your time and energy?

   _____

   _____

3. What are you sacrificing in the process?

   _____

   _____

4. In the table below, categorize the level of resources you have as low, medium, or high:

Resources	Autonomy	Instrumental Support	Emotional Support	Opportunities for Growth
Low				
Medium				
High				

5. If any of your resources are low, what can you do to increase them?

   _____

   _____

much more to the equation. Could the feeling of being overwhelmed stem from within?

Usually, workers have little or no control over their environment, so they attempt to gain control of their situation by placing high demands on themselves. In this next section, we explore the effects of such internal demands on stress at work and what these self-imposed demands stem from.

High Achievers and Unrelenting Standards

Often, we conflate the terms "high achiever" and "high aimer." While a high achiever is someone who has demonstrated success, a high aimer is someone who continually sets ambitious goals and strives for excellence. While the two may overlap, there's a crucial distinction: a high achiever focuses on past accomplishments, while a high aimer is always looking to the future.

High aimers are characterized by their unrelenting standards. They are not satisfied with mediocrity; they constantly push themselves to new heights. This relentless pursuit of excellence often stems from an intrinsic desire to learn and grow. It's a mindset that drives them to seek challenges, embrace failure as a learning opportunity, and persist in the face of adversity. While this drive for excellence is admirable, it can sometimes tip into perfectionism, an extreme form of high aiming.

The Mindset of the Perfectionist

Ambitious people often work very hard to attain their goals. They have an inner drive to prove themselves, to succeed, and to be recognized for their accomplishments. Many of them set the bar very high and will not settle for mediocrity. Even when everyone around them believes their work is exceptional, the high aimers may still not feel satisfied. That is indicative of a perfectionistic mindset.

If you are a perfectionist, you are not perfect. You just want everything you do to be perfect. You may have unrelenting standards such that you feel like nothing you do is good enough. This keeps you striving to do better and do more and can create the opposite effect of what you want.

Some of the biggest problems perfectionists face include a critical inner voice that tells them they are not good enough, a fear of failure, and a tendency toward procrastination. This triangular trap (figure 2.3) is crucial to understanding what drives high aimers who are perfectionists and what can lead them to burn out.

If you do not believe in yourself enough or if you worry so much about what other people think, you will be less likely to take risks. This can lead to procrastination: You put off your efforts until the last minute so that if you do fail, you can save face by saying that you only worked on the project for a short time, and it is not indicative of your actual ability.

Perfection is not attainable. It is an unrealistic standard we set for ourselves, intended to push us to achieve greater and greater results. Precisely because the standards are impossible

Belief of Inadequacy

Procrastination

Fear of Failure

FIGURE 2.3   The Triangular Trap.

to reach, we are setting ourselves up for failure. Ironically, this is what perfectionists fear the most, and that is why this is a cycle of self-sabotage.

Perfectionism takes up tremendous time and energy. While, in some instances, it can lead to increased performance, the satisfaction is transient. Perfectionists are not typically satisfied because they always expect more from themselves. Even when they attain the desired result, they dwell on ways to improve or run ahead to the next challenge rather than take time to celebrate their win.

It is not surprising that perfectionists exhibit such extreme behaviors: They think about life in black and white terms. It is all or nothing. It is either perfect or it is garbage.

I will explore antidotes to perfectionism later in this book.

TABLE 2.2 **Identify Whether You Are Trapped**

1. Does your inner critique make you feel like nothing you do is good enough?
   - ☐ Yes
   - ☐ No

2. Does your fear of failure lead to procrastination?
   - ☐ Yes
   - ☐ No

3. Do you hold yourself to perfectionistic standards?
   - ☐ Yes
   - ☐ No

If you answered yes to any of these questions, you are likely stuck in the Triangular Trap (see figure 2.3). Don't despair. You will find the answers in this book to get you unstuck.

INTERACTIVE ENVIRONMENTAL
AND PERSONAL STRESSORS

The Transactional Model of Stress theorizes that stress is not found in either the person or the environment, but in the interaction between them.[15] In other words, there is the environment, the person's perception of the environment, and the attempts to cope with the stressors that arise.

You and Your Work Environment

In *The Truth about Burnout*, Christina Maslach and Michael Leiter address problematic interactions between the employee and the job environment by looking at six contributors that, if not adequately addressed, can lead to a job-person mismatch. These contributors include excessive workload, low autonomy, lack of acknowledgment, lack of support, poor ethics, and unfair treatment.[16]

When the workload is excessive and you feel like there is too much to do in the allotted time with the resources available to you, you will probably feel anxiety and irritability as you struggle to get the job done. Because you are not able to accomplish it during office hours, you are more likely to stay late or take work home to complete. This over-commitment to your job robs you of personal time, and you end up feeling guilty about not spending enough time with your family or having the necessary personal time. As I will show you later in this book, without proper time for recovery, you will inevitably burn out.

You might feel mismatched with your job if you have too little autonomy. This is usually the case when you feel micromanaged by your boss, which results in a lack of influence and accountability and can leave you feeling powerless and also lead to burnout over time.

When your efforts are left unacknowledged, you feel devalued. If you are not proud of your work or if you are not gaining a sense of purpose from it, you will place more emphasis on external rewards, including money, prestige, and career advancement. If you feel dissatisfied with these rewards, you are more likely to burn out.

The community aspect of work is often overlooked, but it is a crucial component that can make or break your experience on the job. Humans are wired for connection, so if you feel alienated, if you lack support, or if you are surrounded by constant conflict, you will feel frustrated and on edge. Over time, these feelings can build and push you over the edge to unbearable levels of stress.

If your boss is so focused on results and efficiency that you end up acting unethically, you will lose any sense of meaning you might have otherwise gained from your work which will also lead to burn out.

As with any relationship, you want to be treated fairly at work. If, however, you get blamed for aspects of the job outside of your responsibility, get unequal pay, or see others in your company getting ahead by cheating, you will feel disrespected. This negativity will gnaw at you and can eventually lead to burnout.

Julie, a client of mine, experienced unfair treatment at work. The CEO of the company put her in charge of several accounts. Julie's manager had been her peer and then moved up in the company. When Julie went on vacation, her manager went behind her back and contacted one of Julie's accounts attempting to change the contract with the account holder.

When Julie returned to work and found out what happened, she contacted her company's CFO to discuss the financial ramifications of changing her account's contract. On finding out, her manager demanded that she come into his office for a face-to-face meeting. He felt that Julie made him look bad in

TABLE 2.3 **Matching Yourself to Your Job**

1. Check off any of the following that contribute to a poor job match for you:
   - ☐ Excessive workload
   - ☐ Poor autonomy
   - ☐ Lack of acknowledgement
   - ☐ Lack of support
   - ☐ Poor ethics
   - ☐ Unfair treatment
   - ☐ Role ambiguity

2. In the lines below, write down everything that you focus on about your job that isn't working for you. Be sure to include items you've checked off.

   _____

   _____

   _____

   _____

   _____

3. Now rewrite your story by focusing on what is going well and what went well in the past. Include information about challenges you've overcome, good role models you have come across, and what you have learned along the way.

   _____

   _____

   _____

   _____

   _____

front of the company's upper management and was in a rage. Julie, on the other hand, felt that her manager was threatening and condescending to her and had not only neglected to take the time to understand her job responsibilities, but also tried to undermine her work. This made Julie feel a mixture of outrage and loss of confidence.

In addition to the six contributors to a job-person mismatch, you must understand the responsibilities tied to your role.[17] Without such clarity, you are unable to perform adequately. It is not surprising, then, that role ambiguity has also been linked to job burnout.[18]

Perception and Coping

In addition to identifying any mismatches between you and your work environment, you need to explore two additional factors that may contribute to burnout: (1) the perception you hold of your work environment and (2) your coping style.

Returning to the Transactional Model of Stress, your appraisal of any given situation plays a big role in your stress response and works in two stages.[19] The primary appraisal is when you see potential stressors as threatening. You might reflect on past losses, consider future potential harm, or engage in a current situation that feels challenging.

The secondary appraisal is a consideration of coping resources. In other words, if you see the situation as challenging as opposed to threatening, it is easier to deem it something you can handle, and you will be less likely to experience stress. It is when you feel you cannot cope, whether because there is too much on your plate, too little time, or because you lack the necessary skill to undertake the task, that you feel stressed.

When you appraise a situation as threatening or challenging, there are different ways in which you can cope. To better understand how this works, let us examine work through the lens of a relationship. When you feel frustrated in your love relationship, you can easily find fault with your partner. And some of the time, you would be justified in doing so. But even in the cases of a serious breach of trust like an affair, it is typically not so one-sided: the responsibility for the breakdown of the relationship usually lies with both parties.

In these situations, as always, you are faced with several choices. You can bury your head in the sand, convinced that this is "as good as it gets" and keep trudging along. You can look for a quick fix, perhaps finding excitement outside of the relationship to enliven you, or you can dig deep into the problem and seek out solutions.

The first choice is often the easiest in that it requires no change. The problem with doing nothing, though, is that if you are unhappy with your situation, the prospects for improvement are meager.

The second choice, as noted, provides a quick or substitute solution. Rather than focusing on the root cause, you look for a distraction, a shiny new object in which to invest time and interest. This often takes the form of drugs, alcohol, or emotional eating and can lead to addiction and health problems. What you often find is this approach does not have the effect you want because now you are in a bind. You are living a conflicting double life.

The third option, one that requires quite a bit of courage and determination, is to change things around for the long term. Does this option guarantee you will get the results you want? Not entirely. You only have control over yourself. You cannot be sure how your counterpart will behave. But by shifting your mental and emotional framework, you can experience the situation on an entirely different level, regardless of any external changes.

TABLE 2.4 Managing Perceptions

1. Now that you changed your perception of the situation from "threatening" to "challenging," how well do you think you can cope?

    A. It feels beyond my abilities.
    B. I have some ideas but I'm not super confident.
    C. I trust myself to figure this out.
    D. I know exactly how to handle this.

2. If you picked option A, the uncertainty of the situation is likely contributing to your stress. Whom can you approach for support and guidance?

    _____

    _____

    _____

    _____

3. If you picked option B, you might still want to seek out consultation but you might want to take a leap of faith and try your ideas out first. If you have any fears about that, write about them below.

    _____

    _____

    _____

    _____

4. If you picked option C or D, write below what your plan is and then tackle it!

    _____

    _____

    _____

    _____

The same principles apply at work. To be effective, you need to have insight into what led you to burn out. Then, consider what other ways you can look at your situation. When you can see it through a different lens, you can change your feelings about it as well as your coping strategy. In many cases, by examining the problem and seeking solutions, you will reduce your stress level without changing the job environment.

CONCLUSION

Your work environment and your personality, as well as the interaction between the two, can all lead to burnout. When it comes to your environment, the ideal scenario that leads to engagement is where demands and resources are both high, where demands are challenging rather than hindering, and where you have adequate autonomy.

Personal stressors can be minimized by overcoming beliefs of inadequacy, overcoming fears and a tendency to procrastinate, and by not holding yourself to perfectionistic standards. If you find a mismatch between yourself and your work environment, focus on changing your perception and increasing your coping strategies. Of course, if all else fails, find a more fitting setting for your skills and talents.

CHAPTER 3

Recognizing Burnout Signs

We now know that stress results from perception. When you perceive the demands as far exceeding your resources or ability to cope, you feel stressed. If this stress continues to build over time, not only does performance go down but you become depleted of energy and experience burnout.

Burnout can affect you in many ways. Emotionally, you feel discontented when you put in the effort and cannot produce your desired outcome. Maybe you are used to giving so much of yourself but are so worn out that you feel frustrated when you physically cannot do what you want or perform what is expected of you. The excessive stress can lead to impatience. Even when you achieve your goal, you might find that you get less satisfaction from it.

When you are under duress you might be more prone to emotional reactivity, but once you burn out, you are at risk for extreme anxiety, depression, and anger. Because you lack energy, it becomes nearly impossible to manage your feelings. Over time, the emotional rollercoaster can leave you even more drained or bring you to a state of numbness that blunts even positive emotions. Physicians, for example, who are commonly burned out, are often so hopeless about their situation that they were found to be twice as likely to commit suicide as the normal population and more than any other profession.[1]

Physical symptoms of burnout include dizziness, rapid heart-beat, shortness of breath, insomnia, nausea, and chronic fatigue. Because your immune system is compromised, you are more prone to illness. If you are feeling down and exhausted, chances are you are not taking care of your health. You might find that you do not have the energy to exercise or prepare healthy meals. When you are burned out, you are already in a state of depletion. And without taking time to recover, your situation cannot improve.

Cognitive impairments include forgetfulness and poor concentration, which make it even harder to get the job done. This can cause you to lose motivation. Negative thoughts continually surface, especially when you lack a sense of accomplishment from your work. If productivity is crucial to your self-worth, you will feel inadequate. Eventually, you will become apathetic, isolated from others, and even find excuses for why you should skip work.

Because all these effects can feel overwhelming, you will attempt to stay afloat, but simply coping may be a struggle. You might look for a quick fix, something to distract your mind and numb your feelings. If you find yourself reaching for alcohol the first chance you get when you come home, be forewarned. Addiction commonly develops from burnout. You will need to find real solutions to burnout, not merely an escape.

As I highlighted, burnout can impact your emotional, physical, and mental functioning, but there are three main burnout symptoms to be aware of. These include emotional exhaustion, cynicism, and reduced personal accomplishment.

To provide you with a visual depicting the symptoms of burnout, I've created an infographic that you can access on www.BurnoutToResilience.com.

EMOTIONAL EXHAUSTION

Emotional exhaustion is a state of mental fatigue due to an accumulation of stress. People experiencing emotional exhaustion often feel like they have no power or control over what happens in their lives. They may feel "stuck" or "trapped" in a situation. The lack of energy, poor sleep, and decreased motivation they experience can make it even more difficult to overcome the problem. Over time, this chronic, stressed-out state can cause permanent damage to their health.

Karasek's Demands–Control Model of job stress, described in chapter 2, helps us understand what brings about exhaustion. In no uncertain terms, a major cause of emotional exhaustion is a high workload coupled with low autonomy on the job.

High Demands + Low Autonomy
= Emotional Exhaustion

If you are tired all the time, it is likely you are burning out. You put in a long workday, commute home, and then work from home some more. Your work responsibilities are never done, and you feel like you are living to work instead of working to live. There is no time for anything else. When the weekend finally arrives, if you actually find time not to work, you might find that you do not have the energy to do anything fun. You just want to catch up on sleep or veg out in front of the television.

Once you are over "the hump" of emotional exhaustion, subtle signs of stress become more pronounced. Healthy engagement, which enables stress hardiness, becomes over-engagement with high stress levels. There is a heightened sense of urgency and hyperactivity in this frantic state. You intend to invest more of yourself to conquer your task list, but when expectations are too high and time and resources are depleted, you lack the energy required.

While no one wants to burn out, researcher and author Brené Brown points out that exhaustion has become a status symbol.[2] We live in a culture that emphasizes the importance of work and accomplishment. Too often, you can get caught up in overworking and feel proud of self-sacrifices such as skipping lunch or never taking a vacation. When you are adequately tired, this is a sign you are a hard worker, which is culturally admirable.

In reality, if what you care about is accomplishment, you have to think about how to maintain your energy, not drain it, so that you can keep going.

While exhaustion may seem like an easily identifiable symptom to observe, it is often misunderstood and under-appreciated. To find out whether you are indeed exhausted, tune into your energy level. If when you started your job you felt energized and now you are feeling drained to the point that you are dragging yourself around, you are burning out.

Emotional exhaustion is an indication that you need to recover from work-related stress. Some indicators that you are energy-depleted include the inability to relax at the end of the day when you are home. You continue to ruminate about your work and find it hard to focus on personal tasks. Physically you feel tired, and it may take you a couple of days to recover your energy. When you are overly fatigued, you may find that on arriving at home you need to be alone for a while before interacting with others, and you lack the energy to engage in any leisure activity or even engage with your work.

When you are worn out, this can bring a sense of dread about going to work. Not only do you struggle while at the office, but

TABLE 3.1 Exhaustion Inventory

Before you move forward to delve into solutions, find out how exhaustion or other burnout symptoms may be affecting you.

To measure early signs of fatigue at work, consider these items that were adapted from the *Need for Recovery Scale*. Give yourself 10 points for each "Yes" response. Scores fall in a range from 0 to 100. Higher scores indicate a greater need for energy recovery after work.

	Exhaustion Inventory	Yes	No
1.	Toward the end of the workday, does fatigue keep you from being as productive as you usually are?		
2.	Do you feel tired out by the time you leave work?		
3.	Do you have trouble relaxing after work?		
4.	Do you find it hard to show interest in other people when you arrive home?		
5.	When you get home after work, do you need to be left alone for some time?		
6.	After work, does it take over an hour to feel entirely recovered?		
7.	Do you find that after dinner you are still in bad shape?		
8.	Do you feel so tired after work that you lack the energy to engage in leisure activities?		
9.	Is it hard to focus outside of work?		
10.	Does it take two consecutive nonworking days before you can start to relax?		

Total:

also during recovery attempts. It may be hard to fall asleep despite your fatigue. When the energy you need is not restored, your ability to do your job well is undermined and makes it difficult to concentrate and remember critical details.

Passionate people may destroy their relationships or physically pass out from emotional exhaustion but not burn out the way a frazzled worker might. When you are not clicking with your role, when you feel overloaded, and when your duties are not aligned with your expectations or values, it is not merely the stress that gets to you, but you will experience a perspective shift. You will feel like you cannot make progress and consequently disengage and become cynical and pessimistic over time.

CYNICISM

When you are exhausted, you are extremely low on energy. You might feel like things are not working out. Maybe you are trying to do all the things that you typically do but you are not getting the same results. In essence, you go from being effective at your job to being ineffective. It can feel frustrating because it is not that you lack the skills or the know-how; something is getting in the way. This frustration might fuel you to invest even more energy to get the results that you are used to getting, but if that doesn't work, over time, your attitude changes. You go from a place of feeling enthusiastic and excited about your job to feeling cynical. This is when you feel like your work is "just a job."

Cynicism is mentally distancing from work, minimizing engagement, and giving up on ideals. This is an attempt to protect your energy and prevent further disappointment.

TABLE 3.2 **Reversing Defeatism**

When you give up on yourself, it's only a matter of time until you fail. Whether you think you can or can't do your job, you are right.

In the lines below, write about a work situation in which you currently feel cynical about your ability to accomplish a task and why.

_____

_____

_____

_____

_____

Now think about how you can turn this situation around.

_____

_____

_____

_____

_____

If you are working with customers, you might stop seeing them as people with needs and start thinking of them as "just another part of my day I have to get through." This leads to decreased customer service and increased errors, and it can negatively affect how you feel about yourself, especially if you typically take pride in your work. You might feel angry at your company for putting you in this situation or you might feel like you are stuck in a job that brings you no joy or sense of purpose.

In fact, on reaching burnout, you have less capacity for empathy. Coupled with impatience and irritability, this renders you unable to have working relationships with your customers or coworkers.

According to the Job Demands–Control Model (figure 2.2), while high demands lead to exhaustion, low autonomy is what brings about cynicism.[3] This is especially true for workers who struggle with time management and who have few resources with which to work.

When a job is very demanding of your time, energy, and focus, and when you feel like you do not have enough resources to stay afloat, you are likely to push yourself harder and harder. At first you might be successful at getting some projects completed, but soon you will recognize how unsustainable this pattern is and start to feel anxious about how you are going to manage. This anxiety is especially pronounced when you feel as though you are running out of steam.

If you find yourself in this position, turn your anger into a fight for increased support, more resources, and for getting tasks taken off your plate. Over time, however, when you are met with resistance, your anger can turn into a sense of detachment and cause you to feel deflated. You may feel like a lone soldier on the battlefield trying to fight a war that is way over your head. You know it's "mission impossible," but you stick it out and think, "I have to keep going."

If high demands are the equivalent of you drowning, then cynicism is you making it to shore. The shore, however, is that of an island. While on this island, isolation leads you to feel disconnected from others.

You lose your sense of enjoyment at work as you indulge in negative self-talk. Consequently, you look for ways to avoid work by calling in sick more, coming in late, or not answering calls and emails.

REDUCED PERSONAL ACCOMPLISHMENT

Given that burnout leads to reduced capacity for concentrating, decision-making, and overall coping, what might have been easy to do in the past becomes increasingly more difficult. Because operating in a hectic manner is unsustainable, over time you will become disengaged, noticing that despite all efforts you are not accomplishing as much as before.

A sense of helplessness and hopelessness can set in and can negatively affect not only performance and motivation, but the appraisal of performance at work. You may no longer see your work as an opportunity for accomplishment, you may stop believing in your ability to be productive, or you might blame yourself for not being able to keep up. When your mind is filled with negative self-talk, you stop taking risks, thereby accomplishing less, which only reinforces your belief that you "CAN'T do this job."

Journalist Ulrich Kraft discusses a burnout model proposed by psychologists Herbert J. Freudenberger and Gail North, which is composed of 12 stages (figure 3.1).[4]

Stage 1: The cycle begins with a compulsion to prove yourself and is predominantly found in perfectionists.

Stage 2: You are led to work harder because you want to be irreplaceable.

Stage 3: The excessive drive eventually leads you to neglect your needs.

Stage 4: Sleep, meals, and social interactions all become erratic. You become aware that something is wrong, but you don't notice the physical symptoms of stress that are upon you.

Stage 5: In an attempt to adjust to the environment and make it manageable, you revise your values. Everything that is not

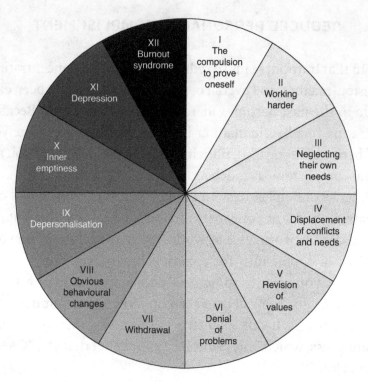

FIGURE 3.1 The Burnout Model. *Source*: Freudenberger and North, *Women's Burnout*.

work-related you deem unimportant, and notions of work-life balance, friends, and family, as well as hobbies are dismissed, all to get the job done.

Stage 6: When problems emerge, you deny them, become cynical, or place blame on the demands of the job and the time-frame rather than the changes that have occurred in your life.

Stage 7: To release the stress, you withdraw by using substances.

Stage 8: You become fearful, apathetic, and experience feelings of worthlessness. You exhibit odd behavioral changes that concern your friends and family.

Stage 9: Your sense of self and ability to tune in to your own needs is lost.

Stage 10: A sense of emptiness sets in, and you become reactive and impulsive. This may lead to an overreaction to situations that feel stressful and to looking for ways to compensate and fill the void through the consumption of excessive food, alcohol, or drugs.

Stage 11: You become depressed and life loses its meaning.

Stage 12: Finally, you are burned out and mentally and physically collapse.

CONCLUSION

Burnout can affect you emotionally, physically, and cognitively. When demands are high, you are more likely to experience emotional exhaustion. When autonomy is low, your attitude about work might turn cynical. When you run out of steam, your performance and, hence, your accomplishments decline.

Life doesn't have to be so grim. Burnout is something that can happen for various reasons and can express itself in various ways, but there are proven systems to overcome burnout as well as prevent it. You're about to uncover seven different strategies to deal with burnout before it's too late.

PART II

Active Practice

Emotional Intelligence

Knowing others is intelligence; knowing yourself is true wisdom.
—LAO TZU, *TAO TE CHING*

In chapters 4 through 10, we will examine the two essential competencies of emotional intelligence, personal and social. You will gain wisdom and power as you improve your personal competency, and you will increase intelligence and strength as you develop your social competency.

Much of what you're about to read is the culmination of the life goals of many of my clients—being productive, self-motivated, and influential. In a word: effective. The following chapters will highlight the skills you will need to develop in order to withstand external obstacles with grace.

Personal Competency

Often, our biggest obstacles include distrust in ourselves or others, being overcome with fear, feeling overwhelmed by stress or anxiety, lacking motivation, and believing we are inadequate. Each of these can be addressed by increasing your emotional intelligence.

Personal competency begins with an understanding of yourself through which you can better manage your reactions. To help you fully grasp the concepts and the associated skills, I have divided this competency into four chapters.

In the first (which is chapter 4 of this book), we will examine how to increase self-awareness. Chapter 5 discusses emotional literacy and examining six of the most common emotions. Chapter 6 looks at how you can use your awareness, self-control, and self-expression to master your emotions. Then, chapter 7 helps you put your skills to use to achieve optimal performance. The idea is that when you know yourself, you can manage yourself better, which leads to better performance results.

Self-Awareness

Emotional Literacy

Emotional Mastery

Optimal Performance

Personal competency.

CHAPTER 4

Self-Awareness

Being self-aware is the cornerstone of emotional intelligence. It is vital to decision-making, to satisfying your needs and desires, to feeling safe and in control, and to living with purpose.

Think about the last time you were at a job interview or on a first date. A question that we often struggle with is, "What can you tell me about yourself?" Sure, this question is vague, very general, and you may not know where to start. Likewise, due to your blind spots, it is a tough question to answer adequately.

There are a variety of ways to increase your self-awareness. We will focus on seven areas to master.

1. KNOW YOUR STRENGTHS AND WEAKNESSES

I recently worked with a client who was feeling burned out at work. She was not even aware she was burned out, but upon reflection on her work history, she noticed a pattern. She would push herself to work hard, but there was a misalignment between what she wanted to focus on and the work she was assigned. After a while, she would quit her job and look for a new one.

I had her take a personality assessment called the Myers-Briggs Type Indicator (MBTI) so we could gain insight into her strengths and weaknesses. Armed with this new information and discussing how her strengths and weaknesses applied to her job, it was easy to see where she could thrive at work and what she needed to leave behind. This conversation inspired her to talk to her manager and feel enthusiastic about changing the course of her job responsibilities.

If you want to be effective, you need to play to your strengths. You also need to know your weaknesses so that you minimize the amount of time and energy you spend on those areas and focus on improving them over time. By understanding and accepting your limitations, you avoid overestimating your abilities and can strategically delegate certain tasks to others whose strengths are more aligned with those areas.

We often have a hard time acknowledging our talents because they are just part of what makes us who we are. But consider this: Let's say that from the age of eight, you spent 30 minutes a day practicing piano. What do you think motivated you to sit down and play every day when you could have been watching television or playing outside? Perhaps it was determination because you believed in your abilities. Are you the kind of person who, once you make up your mind about something, perseveres? If so, how can you use that in the work setting?

Maybe playing the piano was an activity that allowed you to get into a meditative state. When working, what types of activities enable you to get into a state of flow? What are the circumstances that allow you to relax and allow your talents to shine?

When you play cards or board games, do you strategize and think two or three steps ahead of your opponent? If so, how can you apply this ability at work to anticipate what other people want, think, and might do? This is your superpower. Use it wisely.

2. KNOW YOUR PERSONALITY

According to researchers and authors of the MBTI,[1] Isabel Briggs Myers and her mother, Katherine Briggs, one dimension of personality is extroversion-introversion.

Your coping strategy for dealing with stress should be modified based on where you are on this spectrum. For example, you need to set realistic expectations for yourself. If you are an introvert, this means allowing for recovery time from social exchanges because being around others takes its toll. If you are an extrovert, this means seeking out social opportunities when your energy is low because being with others gives you the boost you need.

One of the traps you can fall into is comparing yourself to others. If you are an introvert and see a colleague accepting more social invitations after work, going to one networking event after another, or discussing weekend plans at lunch with the entire team, recognize that they are likely extroverted. Rather than consider yourself inadequate in comparison, focus on the personal strengths that make you unique as an introvert.

If you are an extrovert, you might notice how easily a colleague creates intimate interactions with coworkers or works alone, focusing well without the need for socializing, or generating ideas that seem introspective. Instead of feeling inferior, note that your extroverted tendencies just mean that you have different areas of strength.

3. BE AWARE OF YOUR EMOTIONS

It is easy to know when your car needs gas because the gas gauge serves as a visual reminder. Unfortunately, you do not have a

TABLE 4.1 Increasing Your Self-Knowledge

To know your strengths, weaknesses, and other dimensions of your personality, use the Myers-Briggs Type Indicator (MBTI; available at https:/www.myersbriggs.org) or a free version of a similar instrument (available at https:/www.16personalities.com).

Based on the feedback you get, answer the following questions:

1. What are you good at? When you think about the work you've done in the past, what was easy for you? Perhaps you found yourself able to do something that was a struggle for others around you. If so, what was that? Think back to your past jobs, volunteer positions, and life experiences. What do people compliment you on? Is it your ability to make decisions, your time-management skills, your ability to lead a team, your creative solutions to problems, or some combination?

_____

_____

_____

_____

2. What are your type's stated weaknesses, and how do you see these affecting your work?

_____

_____

_____

_____

3. How can you maximize your strengths and minimize your weaknesses in your job?

_____

_____

_____

_____

visible indicator for your emotions, but even so, you can become more attuned to your feelings.

Emotions are energy that manifests differently in the body depending on the emotion you feel. Close your eyes and scan your body. Where do you feel tension or discomfort? Ask yourself to associate a feeling with that bodily sensation and see what comes up.

Emotions are contagious. Just because you feel something does not mean it belongs to you. Ask yourself, "Who does this stress belong to?" You might realize you have absorbed your partner's or your colleague's stress just by being around them. In that case, focus on letting it go. It is not your stress, and you do not have to hold onto it.

You can also go back in your mind to past experiences. If, for instance, it is hard for you to associate physiological symptoms with angry feelings, bring to mind an experience that made you angry in the past. With your eyes closed and your mind focused, notice what sensations arise. This is how anger manifests for you physically. Consider making a note of that sensation, and next time you feel this way in your body, let it be an indication that you are angry. You can do this for each of the emotions.

The more you are aware of what you are feeling, the more authentically you will come across in conversations. Your body language gives away your true feelings, so being aware of your emotions allows you to be mentally in sync, express your thoughts and feelings accurately, and get your needs met, thereby addressing the issue at hand.

As mentioned earlier, we all have blind spots. Getting feedback from a boss or coach or through leadership assessments helps you understand perceptions others have of you and will shine a light on your behavioral patterns.

TABLE 4.2 Reflecting on Your Emotions

Think back to a time when you felt each of the emotions below and write down how the feeling manifested in your body (e.g., heat, tension, pain).

1. Fear

_____

_____

2. Anger

_____

_____

3. Sadness

_____

_____

4. Guilt

_____

_____

5. Shame

_____

_____

6. Joy

_____

_____

Journaling provides you with an opportunity for self-expression and is something on which you can look back to identify patterns. Meditation is another useful tool. It helps to increase mindfulness, which is an opportunity to delve into yourself to notice and release thoughts, emotions, and bodily sensations. By raising awareness of yourself, you will make more intuitive and fitting decisions.

4. KNOW WHAT YOU NEED AND WANT

Imagine you are driving a vehicle. You need to have a destination in mind. Your goal will determine the destination. If you need to buy milk, you will drive to the grocery store. If you want to visit a friend, you will drive to their house. If you want to combine them, you will figure what route to take so you can buy milk on your way home. By focusing on your needs and desires, you will direct your actions to be purposeful rather than being reactive and wasting your resources.

When you are clear on your needs, you can communicate them to others and increase the likelihood of getting them met. But you may ask, "What is the best way to identify my needs?"

Abraham Maslow talked about needs in terms of a hierarchy or pyramid (figure 4.1).[2]

It makes sense that before you can focus on anything else, you have to meet all of your physiological needs, including food, water, clothing, and shelter. Once you take care of the basics, you can focus on safety and security issues such as employment, money, and health.

Next, you can focus on the need we are all wired for: connection. As human beings, we require love and belonging, and this includes friendship, family, and sexual intimacy.

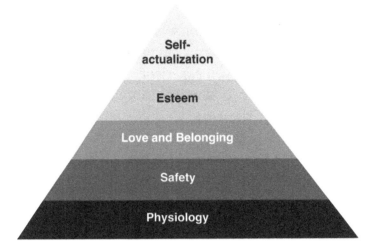

FIGURE 4.1   Maslow's hierarchy of needs. *Source*: Maslow, "A Theory of Human Motivation."

The next level of the pyramid focuses on esteem. This is where we seek ways to feel confident, get the respect of others, and gain a sense of achievement.

Lastly, we reach the highest level: the need for self-actualization. According to Maslow, we are self-actualized when we behave morally, use our creativity, can be spontaneous, can problem-solve, and accept the facts. When it comes right down to it, this need is when the right and left sides of our brain are working together to bring logic in touch with our feelings so we can flourish. You will read more about the hierarchy of needs in chapter 14.

You can tune into your emotions to better understand your needs. If, for instance, you are feeling angry, this is an indication one or more of your needs are not being met. Ask yourself, "What do I need to turn down the dial on my anger?" Further, to be accurately attuned, you need to differentiate between primary and secondary emotions.

Anger is a secondary emotion, which means that there is another feeling underneath it. Anger is the feeling you have about your primary feeling, and it can intensify long past the triggering event. The patterns you experience may go back to childhood, so if the anger feels familiar, it may be a long-stemming way of interacting in the world.

To understand how you truly feel, rather than being reactive, first find out what might be beneath the anger. Are you lonely, sad, or afraid? Once you identify the primary emotion, you need to deal with it rather than mask or avoid it. This reduces the emotion's intensity and allows you to powerfully cope with situations as they present themselves.

Each emotion connects to a thought. While you have tens of thousands of thoughts per day, you will need to do some detective work to find the notion that relates most closely to your emotion. Then notice whether the thought is about something or someone else. If it is, you will need to dig deeper to identify what your belief is about yourself.

Let's say, for example, that someone at work confronts you about the way you handled a procedure. When you think back on the incident now, you recognize that you were upset about the confrontation and were defensive in your response. In hindsight, you might be aware that you tend to one-up others in situations like these.

This is where you will need to get curious to figure out the unmet need. When you reflect on your life, what is the motivation that leads you to try to prove yourself right during conflicts? Maybe it's because you worry that others will not take you seriously. If that is your perception, what would it mean about you if this were true? You might believe that you are not important. Your need might therefore be to feel significant and heard.

TABLE 4.3 **Familiarizing Yourself with Your Needs**

Take a look at Maslow's hierarchy of needs (figure 4.1) and note below where on the pyramid your main needs lie at the moment.

_____

_____

_____

Identify the emotion that best represents how you currently feel about your situation at work.

_____

_____

_____

What is the unmet need beneath this emotion?

_____

_____

_____

Once you recognize your need, you might consider more effective ways of meeting it.

5. KNOW YOUR TRIGGERS

Triggers are emotional overreactions you have to circumstances happening now that have roots in one or more events from your past.

You might notice that every time you drive by a place where you used to work, you feel nauseous. Perhaps when your friend arrives late to your dinner date, you find yourself panicking about her safety. If you are hypervigilant even when walking down a very safe street, this fear is an overreaction.

Saying that you are overreacting is not a judgment, but an observation. If you consider the situation and your reaction to it objectively, and if you realize the two are not congruent, chances are you feel triggered.

You may have a perfectly good reason to react the way you do. The old workplace may have left an emotional scar, making it challenging to be around without reliving old memories. If at one time someone you waited for did not show up because something terrible happened to them, you will likely remember that story each time you are waiting for someone. And if you have ever been accosted while walking outside or heard of a physical attack happening to someone else, it might trigger you to be extra vigilant whenever you walk alone.

Neurobiologist R. Douglas Fields identified that our triggers usually fall into one of nine categories.[3] He came up with the acronym LIFEMORTS to capture these trigger types:

- Life or death: These are survival-based triggers, like the example of being hypervigilant while walking alone outside. You are trying to protect yourself from harm.

- Insults: When someone hurls a hurtful phrase at you and degrades your integrity, you might feel triggered. When this happens, you might become angry and try to defend yourself. It may lead to rumination and to internalizing the insult, which can result in having other feelings, such as depression.

- Family: This refers to protecting family members from danger.

- Environment: Protecting your home is an example of an environmental trigger. It is also imperative to your survival.

- Mate: You might be triggered when there is a threat against your mate because you want to keep them safe.

- Order in society: Perceiving a social injustice happening to yourself or others can be triggering.

- Resources: This refers to obtaining and protecting resources such as money. When something threatens your resources, you might become triggered.

- Tribe: When the group you identify with (e.g., your country or religion) is negatively affected, you might also feel adversely affected.

- Stopped: You may feel triggered as a result of being prevented from pursuing what you want. Examples include imprisonment or being physically cornered.[4]

The more you know your triggers, the more you will be able to avoid triggering situations that put you at risk for an extreme emotional reaction or at least to prepare yourself in advance. Conversely, by identifying what you are avoiding, you will be able to familiarize yourself with your triggers and use that information to prepare for facing challenges.

6. GET IN TOUCH WITH YOUR VALUES

We all seek meaning in our lives. When we are clear about what we value, we can direct our decisions and behaviors to be more

TABLE 4.4 **Finding Your Triggers**

Identify your triggers in each of the LIFEMORTS areas that is applicable.

- Life or death:

  _____

  _____

- Insults:

  _____

  _____

- Family:

  _____

  _____

- Environment:

  _____

  _____

- Mate:

  _____

  _____

- Order in society:

  _____

  _____

- Resources:

  _____

  _____

- Tribe:

  _____

  _____

- Stopped:

  _____

  _____

  What can you learn from your triggers to protect your energy?

  _____

  _____

purposeful. Do not let ego get in the way of your decisions. Instead, be true to yourself and others.

When you know your values, you can optimize your environment. This is key to avoiding burnout. If you are a doctor, for instance, you might consider whether you prefer a fast-paced work environment where you expend energy throughout the day (e.g., an emergency room setting) or a slower-paced environment that focuses on relationship building (e.g., a health clinic). Your values can shape your preferences and inform your decisions.

One value that determines how I live my life is balance. I love my work, I love my family, and I love my time alone. To feel complete, I have designed my life so that there is time for each of these aspects.

When you are not intentional about creating your experiences based on your values, you can easily fall out of balance, primarily if you are focused on only one aspect of your life, such as your career. You will learn more about values in chapter 33.

7. KNOW YOUR BELIEFS

We all identify with our story. It is our personal history, our collection of memories and early experiences that have shaped the way we see ourselves and others around us. What is your story? What beliefs do you hold as a result of your early life experiences? The more in touch you are with your beliefs, the more you will see how they affect your interpretation of events, your feelings, and your decisions.

For example, my client Tammy showed up to our session upset the week after Mother's Day. Her father, with whom she had a problematic relationship, had sent her a package of hats as a Mother's Day gift. These were hats he had received as free giveaways. Tammy was upset because she interpreted the gesture as an indication that she was not important enough to him to actually buy a gift. Meanwhile, her husband asked her why she had not thanked her father and threw out the hats.

Tammy and her husband had different reactions to the same event because they had different upbringings and associated beliefs. The reason Tammy had the reaction she did was that she has been carrying around a belief since childhood that her father does not think she is important. Our brains try to find evidence to justify our ideas. In this case, Tammy was able to associate the "thoughtless" gift with her importance.

Throughout our work, Tammy was able to widen her lens— which is an essential aspect of changing personal stories. The more she thought about it, the more she realized that, in fact, her father was the only person who had given her a Mother's Day gift at all. While the hats were not what she wanted, she was able to recognize that the contents were not a reflection of her. Instead, they were a reflection of her father, who liked to

TABLE 4.5 **Identifying Your Limiting Beliefs**

Check the boxes beside any of the limiting beliefs that apply to you.

☐ My needs won't be met.

☐ I can't be successful.

☐ I can't control myself.

☐ Other people's needs are more important than my own.

☐ I have to stay vigilant/perfect or something terrible will happen.

☐ There is something wrong with me.

☐ I am not enough.

☐ Other people cannot be trusted.

☐ I don't belong with other people.

☐ I can't do my work without other people's help.

☐ I am a failure.

☐ I am better/smarter than anyone else around me.

☐ I care more about people's perception of me than about being authentic.

☐ If others knew how I feel, they wouldn't like me or they would judge me.

☐ When people make mistakes, they should pay the price.

☐ Other:

---

collect free samples and wanted to share them as a thoughtful token.

Through the process of changing your story, you can change your state of mind. Therapy is one of the best avenues to help you identify and overcome limiting beliefs. I cannot overstate the importance of this work. It allows you to get beyond your stuck points, which start in your mind. Noticing triggers and working through them is an opportunity to break old patterns, whether in behaviors or relationships with others.

CONCLUSION

Being aware of yourself is very important. It serves as the basis on which one builds self-mastery. When you do not know yourself or what is driving your emotions and needs, you will not be your best self and can easily take on the identity other people want you to have. This leaves you feeling empty inside.

Self-awareness is a work in progress. It requires you to continually check in with yourself and notice what is happening within you. Assessing your strengths and weaknesses, personality, needs, triggers, values, and beliefs is a start, as these are typically stable over time. From there, you can focus on your emotions, which will be affected daily and change throughout each day. Once you are equipped with self-knowledge, you can begin to manage your reactions and be more in control.

CHAPTER 5

Emotional Literacy

We learn about ourselves through self-reflection and mindfulness. Given this knowledge, we can direct our energies to gain control over our reactions and thereby accomplish more and feel better about ourselves. In honing our self-competence skills, we gain true wisdom and power.

Awareness is always the first step to creating change. We have to be aware of what aspects of our lives make us unhappy, draw motivation to change them, and then exert effort consistently over time to see results.

But simply being aware is not sufficient. As the Buddhist proverb says, "To know and not to do is not to know." We must take the knowledge we have gained and use it for self-mastery.

There is a Buddhist tale about two monks about to cross a rushing stream. They are approached by a beautiful young woman who asks if they would carry her across, so she won't get wet and have to endure the cold temperature of the water. The young monk was disgusted by her request. He ignored her and crossed the stream alone. The old monk picked her up, carried her across and set her down on the other side. The woman thanked the monk and went on her way. The two monks continued down the road.

The young monk continued to be furious. At first he was silent, but after a while, when he could not hold back any longer, he finally exploded. He yelled at his companion for carry-ing the woman stating, "You know it is forbidden for monks to touch women!"

In response to the young monk's anger, the older monk said, "Oh, no! Are you still carrying that woman? I put her down an hour ago."

We have all had instances where we got swept away by a strong emotion. Life can feel stressful and overwhelming at times, and it is easy to succumb to such experiences by crum-bling or letting the feelings build inside us until we explode. We have to manage our emotions the way a tightrope walker main-tains their balance. These artists must perfect their craft, fo-cusing solely on biomechanics. They must be present in mind and emotionally calm.

To truly master your feelings, you must first understand them. Here are six of the most common emotions we experi-ence regularly.

FEAR

Our survival instinct kicks into gear when we believe we are threatened. Our body produces adrenaline and goes into what is known as a *fight or flight* response. We become energized in the face of danger to either fight off the threat or remove our-selves from the perceived danger.

While this response is appropriate and vital when we are in-deed in harm's way, the majority of our fear lives in our mind, not in any physical reality. Our brain has not adapted from the time we were cave dwellers to know the difference.

Fear is associated with stress and anxiety. When we are afraid, we experience a stress response and have anxious thoughts about the future. Stress is an experience we have based on our interpretation of events. A testament to this is when an event takes place, each person's reaction to that same event is different. This is because we view the event through a lens shaped by our life experiences.

So the next time you notice your heart fluttering, your head swimming with anxious thoughts, and your breathing as shallow, remind yourself that you are safe. Gaining perspective on the situation can help calm you down so you can focus on problem-solving.

What you need most to act in the face of fear is courage. Without it, you feel dis*courage*d. Having the support of others will give you the confidence you need to feel en*courage*d to take action.

ANGER

We often feel angry when faced with an injustice, like when someone falsely accuses us of an act we did not commit or when we feel disrespected by others. When anger sets in, you might notice your temperature rising. Anger creates heat inside of us, and if we do not manage our anger properly, it will reach its boiling point, and we will likely explode.

Rather than think of yourself as a pressure cooker, someone who lets resentment build and build over time, it is best to notice when you begin to feel upset and take immediate charge of the situation.

One way to do this is by paying attention to your language. Have you ever dismissed someone's compliment of you? If it is possible to keep positive influences out due to our determination to deflect praise, we can say the same about negativity.

Make up your mind that others' criticisms and judgments have no influence on your mood.

Daniel J. Siegel, an American neuropsychiatrist, coined the phrase "Name it to tame it," explaining that by naming your emotion, you can begin to gain mastery over it.[1] The other piece to consider is what to call your emotional experience. The richer your vocabulary of emotional terms, the easier it will be to intervene.

Let's say your manager promised to meet with you each Friday at noon to go over your weekly progress and discuss upcoming projects. Somehow, as you get to the end of the week, you notice that your manager has a completely booked schedule. He bumps your meeting off until next week. The following week he is 20 minutes late. The week after that, he tells you he has to leave early. You value these meetings as they are part of your plan for getting a promotion. You tell yourself that if you aren't able to have face-to-face time with your manager, you will likely stay stuck in your current position.

After the first occurrence of neglect, you feel frustrated but try to stay optimistic and maybe even understanding of your manager's busy schedule. The next time he brushes you off, you feel annoyed. By the third time he cancels your meeting, you are furious.

By naming your emotions, you can see where on the spectrum you are. By using different labels such as "frustrated," "annoyed," and "furious," you stay aware of the intensity of your emotions.

The more an injustice takes place over time, the more we go from irritated to enraged. The danger is that when we escalate emotionally, our rational brain goes offline. It becomes harder and harder to control our behaviors, and we are more prone to overreacting by saying or doing something we will likely regret.

Instead, we need to intervene sooner by asserting ourselves. In the above scenario, you might firmly remind your manager how significant you find these weekly meetings and check in to see what is getting in the way of him making it a priority.

Anger, as previously stated, is a secondary emotion. While it is true that we are angered when someone crosses our personal boundary, underneath that anger is typically another feeling. In some instances, anger is an externalization of our sadness. By getting angry, we become energized to make a change rather than becoming deflated and immobilized.

Alternatively, anger can also be a mask for fear. Being unable to meet with your manager may be infuriating if you are afraid of staying stuck in your position when what you desire is an upward career move. By understanding what you are feeling and how deeply you are feeling it, you can take proactive steps to recover.

SADNESS

We experience sadness whenever there is a loss in our lives. Examples may include losing a loved one or a job, making a geographical move, or experiencing disappointment when reality does not match our expectations. Sadness forces us to slow down physically and mentally. We tend to become sluggish and have a hard time focusing our minds. It is essential to take time to grieve as a way of releasing these feelings. One way we do that is through tears. They shed the pent up anguish we feel and cleanse us from the inside out.

Children have a much easier time releasing their sadness than do adults. Stigmas do not inhibit children. When they experience a loss, they easily cry about it. As we age, we learn that crying is not socially accepted. In a work setting, it is often considered unprofessional. Many cultures deem crying a sign of weakness. This belief contributes to the stigma of emotional expression.

There is a fine line between expressing our feelings in a healthy way and being out of control. When we push our feelings down, we become numb. The tricky thing about this phenomenon is that when we numb our feelings in one realm, we become numb in other realms as well. So, when you don't allow yourself to feel sadness, for example, you will also become numb to joy.

The key is to find healthy outlets for your feelings and to express yourself assertively, so you meet your needs. That way, you can stay emotionally balanced.

GUILT

Our moral code is something we develop through family and cultural norms. We are taught right from wrong and then add our interpretations of what we should and should not do.

It is when we believe we have crossed our moral line in the sand that we feel guilty. The purpose of this emotion is to remind us of our rule to keep us in line.

There are two optimal ways to handle guilt. One is to learn from your mistakes, so you do not step out of line again. It might include repenting for your actions, as in asking for forgiveness. It is righting your wrong.

Other times, you might feel guilty for having an antiquated rule in place that no longer fits. Now that you have changed your way of thinking, you feel guilty for not sticking to your original method of doing things. In that case, ask yourself a simple question, "Does this rule still make sense for me?" Rather than being loyal to an outdated rule, you have an opportunity for revision.

Once you take action by either learning from your immoral act or changing your moral code, you can release the guilt. It has served its purpose.

SHAME

Of all the emotions we experience, shame is the only one that does not help us in any way. Unlike guilt, where you believe you have done something wrong, shame is the belief that there is something wrong with you.

It is easy to see why you may feel shame. Growing up, you may have heard adults say, "You should be ashamed of yourself." Shame is other people's way of controlling you, and when you hear it enough from others, you internalize it. You start to believe that there is something wrong with you, that you are not enough.

From all my years of professional experience, I have found that many of the problems we face internally boil down to a feeling of inadequacy. We often lack confidence, suffer from chronic self-doubt, and fear failure because of internalized shame.

When you recognize shame in yourself, ask yourself whether it is related to an immoral behavior—in which case you can substitute guilt—or to a belief that there is something fundamentally wrong with you. If the latter rings true, investigate the origin of this belief and any evidence for it. Then consider the aspects of your character that are positive. If you were to ask your loved ones why they care so much about you, what would they say? We are often so harsh on ourselves that we omit evidence contrary to our beliefs even though it is staring us straight in the face. To achieve a balanced perspective, we must consider both sides.

JOY

The underlying goal we all have in common is the desire to experience joy. I often ask my clients what they want most in life. While for some people it is evident that they want to be happy, many others focus on achievement or material possessions. The quest is to dig deeper and ask why you want what you want. When you dig deep enough, what typically will surface is the desire to feel joy. There is nothing beyond it in the line of questioning. It is our biggest wish.

One of the emotions that gets in the way of joy is guilt. When you believe that you do not deserve to experience joy, you block yourself from pleasure. Some people tend to put others' needs ahead of their own and will sacrifice their happiness as a way to feel important. Having a sense of purpose is vital, but it does not have to be at the expense of joy. Ideally, you can find a way to experience joy and attain a sense of purpose. It is not impossible. It is a state of mind.

CONCLUSION

To engage in the world in an emotionally intelligent way, you must begin the journey with yourself. Pay close attention so you can know yourself, and then make use of that knowledge to manage your own emotions.

Self-management is a skill that requires you to examine your beliefs and challenge your perspectives. By understanding the

TABLE 5.1 Emotional Understanding

In the exercises below, consider your relationship to the six major emotions mentioned in this chapter.

- Fear: What things scare you, and what can you do to lean into your fear?

  _____

  _____

- Anger: What resentments or grudges do you carry, and how does holding onto them affect you?

  _____

  _____

- Sadness: What losses have you experienced about which you feel continually depressed or numb?

  _____

  _____

- Guilt: What do you feel most guilty about? What lessons can you glean from this?

  _____

  _____

- Shame: Identify areas of your life where you feel shame. Would it be appropriate to substitute guilt here instead? Whose voice is shaming you? Is it your inner critic? If so, who does that remind you of in your life?

  _____

  _____

- Joy: Do you believe you deserve to feel joy? If so, do you behave accordingly or do you put other people's needs ahead of your own? If not, identify the belief that is blocking you.

  _____

  _____

purpose of each emotion and by expanding your emotional vocabulary, you can more accurately name what you are feeling. This practice helps decrease the emotional intensity you feel. With the knowledge of what you are feeling and how deeply you are feeling it, you can take proactive steps to recover.

You must look for healthy outlets for your feelings, examine your moral code when guilt gets triggered, focus on what you can control, and remember that ultimately you want to have purpose and to feel joy.

CHAPTER 6

Emotional Mastery

Malcolm Gladwell made popular the notion that with 10,000 hours of practice, usually over a period of 10 years, we attain mastery.[1] Emotional mastery, thankfully, does not have to take that long. It is more about creating daily habits and repetition over time than it is about years of experience.

Despite all your training and good intentions, it is still likely you will have a strong reaction every once in a while. You are engaging in an emotionally intelligent way as long as you stay mindful of what triggers you, how you react to certain events, and what you can take away from an experience to minimize your reaction the next time around.

In this chapter we will explore three aspects of emotional mastery—namely, awareness, self-control, and self-expression. Within each of these areas I have highlighted specific practices you can adopt to strengthen your sense of mastery. You do not, by any means, need to engage in all of these behaviors to reap the benefits. Instead, review the suggestions and find the methods that work best for you.

We will focus on anxiety throughout, as it is the emotion most closely related to burnout. Before we delve in, you need to truly understand anxiety.

Anxiety is an experience you have when you have to do something that scares you or when you worry about something bad happening. But contrary to popular belief, anxiety is not necessarily bad for you.

Think of anxiety on a scale of 1 to 10, with 1 being a state of no anxiety, which you might experience when you are completely Zen or in peaceful sleep, and 10 being when you are in the midst of a panic attack. If 5 is the midpoint, anything below that number can be considered a motivating factor. If you have minimal anxiety, you will likely be lazy as opposed to taking responsibility. Thus, having some anxiety helps motivate you to do the things you need to do. When your anxiety goes above the midpoint, you start to feel distressed and will see a decline in functioning and handling of responsibilities. Too much anxiety impedes your ability to do what it is you need to do (figure 6.1).

Anxiety shows up when you interpret your circumstances as threats, especially when you do not believe you can adequately cope. This usually incorporates a lot of "what if" thinking. What if I miss my flight? What if I lose my job? What if I get lost? What if I show up and don't know anyone? Your brain and body prepare you for facing a life-threatening situation when, in fact, you will make your flight, keep your job, find your way, or are just going to a social event. Overkill, right?

In the words of Corrie Ten Boom, "Worrying is carrying tomorrow's load with today's strength–carrying two days at once.

FIGURE 6.1   Anxiety and functioning.

It is moving into tomorrow ahead of time. Worrying doesn't empty tomorrow of its sorrow, it empties today of its strength."[2]

When you create these negative scenarios in your mind, actually seeing yourself missing your flight and being late to your meeting, you may neglect to notice the physiological manifestations of your anxiety in the body. Anxiety is physiological arousal, so when you feel anxious, the physiology in your body changes. As you will see, there is usually an external circumstance that triggers an innate response.

Physiological symptoms of anxiety can bring up a state of alarm. When you notice something happening in your body that you do not understand or know how to control, this can create even more anxiety.

In the following section you will find approaches to identifying your anxiety and dealing with it effectively.

AWARENESS

The first thing you want to be aware of is how anxiety manifests for you in your body. For each person, it will be a little different. There are a wide variety of symptoms, so just notice what happens for you. When you are feeling anxious, is your mind racing? Do you feel dizzy and faint? Is your heart beating fast? Do you have butterflies in your stomach? Are you sweating? What is happening to you when you are feeling highly anxious at work? Take note. That way, you can become familiar with your pattern and prepare yourself, or at least know that when you feel it, you have a name for it.

You need to identify your work-related triggers. Is it the way that somebody looks at you? Is it a tone of voice? Is it a dynamic between you and other coworkers? What triggers you the most?

You can ready yourself for future scenarios by looking at past triggering episodes.

You are more likely to experience anxiety when you either lack the skills to deal with the situation or lack the confidence to utilize your skills. If, for instance, you are feeling overwhelmed or have too much on your plate, your anxiety might be related to poor time management. Alternatively, if work is placing

---

TABLE 6.1 **Coping with Anxiety**

How does anxiety manifest in your body?

_____

_____

What triggers an anxiety response in you?

_____

_____

Which coping skills might you benefit from working on (e.g., time management, assertive communication) to reduce your anxiety?

_____

_____

What can help you feel more confident to use the coping skills you have?

_____

_____

Do the people you surround yourself with struggle with anxiety? If so, how does that affect you?

_____

_____

unrealistic demands on you, there might be a need for asserting yourself. This includes letting your boss or whoever is delegating you the excessive work know that the expectations are not realistic. You may need to revisit what your responsibilities are for that job.

Lastly, consider how your environment affects you. Moods, we said, are contagious. If the people around you are anxious and you start to feel similarly anxious, recognize that this anxiety may not be your own. In such a case, it would be best to surround yourself with individuals who are more mindful and in control of their emotions.

SELF-CONTROL

Having control over your emotions and, thus, your behavioral response requires you to build up the skills of tolerance and discipline. Once you become aware of your emotional state, you need to be able to ride the wave of your emotions. Knowing that feelings come and go and mindfully noticing what is happening within you rather than becoming fearful or overwhelmed will help you stay calm. The alternative is suppressing the emotion, which is a form of avoidance. While avoidance as a coping strategy may distract you from an unpleasant experience at the moment, it is not a long-term solution. Suppressed emotions tend to get stored in the body and can result in physical pain or autoimmune diseases and eventually rupture in emotional outbursts.

To gain mastery over any area of knowledge or skill, you need an investment of time and energy. What can get in the way of mastery is either boredom or a preference to engage in pleasurable activities.

Imagine that you want to write a book. This requires thought, research in some cases, and many hours of writing and editing. While you have good intentions to sit down and write, you may become distracted by a television show or feel tempted to go out with friends for fear of missing out on the fun. All this temptation causes distraction and procrastination and prevents you from making strides toward your goal. Mastery requires discipline and a delay of instant gratification.

What this has to do with emotional intelligence (EQ) is that your behaviors are a result of your emotional state. If the reason you are procrastinating or giving up on your goal is that you are bored with the repetition of your work, you need to manage your boredom to stick with the task long enough to master it. Similarly, if you are blowing off your commitments to engage in fun, you need to manage your mindset, remember the benefits you will reap in the long run, and set up rewards for milestones along the way. This keeps you moving ahead and will lead to a sense of purpose in your life, which will outlive any short-term gratification you could attain in this moment.

It is not only when you're bored that you seek stimulation and forego possible long-term goals. If you experience low frustration tolerance, this may drive you to impulsivity in many situations. A standard illustration of this is on the road when a person becomes impatient with other drivers, red lights, or pedestrians who cause traffic to slow down. When they act out impulsively, they increase their own risk of being in an accident and hurting themselves and others.

Being aware of how impatient you feel and then taking some deep breaths can help to get your rational brain back online, just when your emotional brain is taking over. Infusing your frustrating moments with relaxation can improve your mindset and sometimes mean the difference between life and death.

TABLE 6.2 Replacing Avoidance or Suppression with Tolerance and Discipline

1. Identify boredom triggers:
   - What tasks do you tend to avoid or procrastinate on?
   - How do you typically cope with boredom (e.g., distraction, avoidance)?

   _____

   _____

   _____

2. Set clear goals and milestones:
   - List your top three goals.
   - Break down each goal into smaller, achievable milestones.
   - Reward yourself for reaching each milestone.

Goals	Milestone 1	Reward 1	Milestone 2	Reward 2

3. Manage impulsive behavior:
   - Reflect on past situations where you acted impulsively due to frustration.
   - Develop strategies to calm down and respond thoughtfully in similar situations.

   _____

   _____

   _____

Set your intention on building up your tolerance of negative feelings and on having the discipline to delay gratification so you can reach your ultimate goals. There is a time and place for everything.

Although you don't have direct access to your emotions, you can manipulate your feelings through your thoughts and behaviors. I have included several cognitive and behavioral strategies below to help you attain a greater sense of control over your emotions.

Cognitive Strategies

We experience anxiety when we think about a future event in a worrying way. Therefore, we should consider various methods to change our thinking to lower our anxiety. We also feel anxious when we experience a failure of sorts and catastrophize what this will mean moving forward. To this end, we will explore cognitive solutions focused on what to do before, during, and after an event.

BEFORE

If you are finding it difficult to make progress, it is likely because you are overthinking things. When you indulge in "what if" thinking, you anticipate everything that might go wrong. By focusing on potential problems, you remain stuck in anxiety. Instead, you need to focus on a solution. You also need to visualize what the worst-case scenario might look like and what you would do if you were in such a dire situation. Allow yourself to quickly figure out what you would do if this were to happen. With your preparation for the worst, you can handle anything less.

As you prepare to move ahead, you need to manage your expectations. When you build up expectations in your mind about the outcomes you want, you can become highly disappointed. These situations can lead to sadness, fear, or anger. Accept that you will face failures as well as successes. Keep in mind the goal you want to attain and stay focused on making headway, even if it means having to change your approach along the way.

DURING

When an intense emotion such as anxiety absorbs you, it might be hard to step out of it enough to apply any intervention. This is where mindfulness is helpful. Once you are mindful of your experience of anxiety or another challenging emotion, you can ask yourself, "On a scale of 0–10, how strongly do I feel this negative emotion?"

Negative emotions are an indication that something is out of alignment. If you are experiencing negativity, you want to do something to change your state. If the intensity is a 7 or above, you want to focus on de-escalation. The goal is to bring the intensity down to a 6 or below. A quick way of doing this is through breathwork. For a visual guide on breathwork, go to my website, www.BurnoutToResilience.com.

Recognize that your feelings result from your thinking. Negative emotions, therefore, result from skewed and unhelpful thoughts. Once you are in control enough, start applying some state-altering interventions. Consider doing a mental inventory of evidence for and against your thoughts. This will widen your lens of the situation and assess for accuracy.

What you experience is not necessarily the truth; it is just your version of the truth, which will likely be different from other people's versions. When the negative emotion you feel is associated with your thoughts of another person, you need to do some reality testing.

In her Netflix documentary *The Call to Courage*, Brené Brown demonstrates a useful technique to check in with others.[3] It asks you to put your interpretation of an event in the context of something your brain made up, which gives you the opportunity to reality test with the other person. If Tammy, who received what she considered to be a thoughtless gift from her father, were to apply this method, she would call her father and say something like, "The story that my brain is making up when I look at the contents of what you sent me is that I am not important." This would allow her father to explain his intention and how he cares very much about her.

Events happen around you continually. Your interpretation of these events leads you to feel the way you do. If your emotions emerge from a thought in your mind, by changing your unhelpful thought to a more helpful one, you can alter your emotional state.

To change your unhelpful thought, use the 3Cs method, which comes from Cognitive Behavioral Therapy.[4] This is a three-step process to help deal with worries, catastrophes, or negative interpretations of events that are causing anxiety.

Step 1: Catch it. What are you thinking about? This is where you identify the thought that is leading to anxiety.

Step 2: Check it. Is this thought accurate? Even if it is valid, is it helpful for you to think this way? Consider how you want to feel. If this thought is causing anxiety and you want to feel calm, it is not helpful. When an idea is either inaccurate or unhelpful, go on to Step 3.

Step 3: Change it. Change your thought to a more accurate one (rather than one based on false information your mind makes up) or to a helpful idea (one that makes you feel how you would prefer to feel).

TABLE 6.3 Cognitive Strategies for Increasing Self-Control

The next time you catch yourself worrying about what might go wrong, stop yourself and substitute the following exercise.

On a scale of 0–10, how anxious do you feel? _____

If you scored 8 or above, focus on taking cleansing breaths until your anxiety goes down to 7 or below. Then proceed with any of the following:

Visualize the worst case-scenario and write it below.

_____

_____

Now consider what you would do to solve the problem should this worst-case scenario really happen and write it below.

_____

_____

Identify the belief(s) that is (are) creating your anxiety. In the table below, list evidence for the belief being true in column 2 and evidence that goes against your belief in column 3.

Belief	Evidence for	Evidence against

Our thoughts can significantly impact our emotions and behaviors. The 3 Cs technique is a powerful tool to manage these thoughts. First, we'll *identify* our thoughts, paying attention to the automatic thoughts that pop into our minds.

Next, we'll *evaluate* these thoughts, determining whether they are helpful or harmful. Finally, we'll *reframe* any negative thoughts into more balanced and realistic ones.

Catch the thought: _____

Check the thought (helpful or unhelpful)? _____

Change the thought to a more helpful one: _____

Is this a situation over which you have control (Y/N)?

If not, focus on letting go of control and accepting the situation.

AFTER

Only certain aspects of the road ahead are in your control. The things you cannot control you need to accept. Learn from and continually adapt to your environment. This is especially important when things do not go your way. Keep things in perspective, and do not allow one disappointment to ruin your mood and spoil the entire day.

Behavioral Strategies

You may recall a time when you became very emotional and impulsively reacted to a situation. This is often the case when you are driving a vehicle. Someone cuts you off or does something that either triggers a thought of being disrespected or a fear of being unsafe, and you become angry and lash out.

Regulating your emotions is about creating a space between the external event and your response to it. In the road rage example, it might be as simple as taking a deep breath or reminding yourself that the other driver's behavior is not a personal attack against you. When you take steps in the moment to slow down your reaction time or to challenge your automatic negative thoughts, you are gaining control of yourself.

You may experience strong negative emotions when something goes wrong and other people are involved. It is vital that you take responsibility for your part rather than focus on shaming or blaming the other person. Instead, you can request that they behave in a way that is preferable to you, but remember that ultimately it is not their behavior that is causing your distress. Rather, it is your thinking about their behavior that is distressing you.

It's always wisest to focus on what you want and how to make it happen, rather than focus on what you don't want. If, for example, your partner seems disengaged at a party, rather than judging, shaming, or feeling frustrated, focus on re-engaging them. By taking action, you are moving toward your goal rather than staying stuck in thought.

Because anxiety is associated with several physiological responses, it is necessary to have a strategy for managing anxiety in the body. Panic is the epitome of anxiety, and it can include a pounding heartbeat, sweating, shaking, dizziness, feeling out of your body, or nausea. If anxiety is an emotion you struggle with often, build up your immunity in advance. Practice relaxation

---

TABLE 6.4 Behavioral Strategies for Increasing Self-Control

- Create a space between the event and your response by taking five deep breaths or counting to 10.
- Take responsibility for your part of the situation.
- Assert yourself if you experience negative feelings due to someone's behavior toward you.
- Practice relaxation daily to build up your immunity to stress.
- Ground your energy when you feel anxious.

every day to prepare your mind and body for dealing with stressful situations as they arise.

Grounding practices are a great way to immediately shift the energy in your body when you are feeling anxious. There are many ways to ground, including walking in nature, lying on the floor, and standing with two feet firmly on the ground while imagining you are a tree sending roots into the earth.

SELF-EXPRESSION

Emotional mastery is not just about self-control. It is also about self-expression. What you are aiming for here is to get your needs met. You must first understand yourself and use this knowledge to be proactive in communicating to others about your experience.

In an online study, researchers examined responses to an EQ test taken by 1,324 people.[5] The data distinguished between responders who were able to apply both self-control and self-expression and those who managed to control their emotions but were unable to talk about their experiences with others.

TABLE 6.5 Increasing Self-Expression

- Pay attention to your inner dialogue.
- Name your inner critic.
- Recognize that your inner critic is trying to help.
- Practice self-acceptance and forgiveness.
- From a place of self-awareness and compassion, assert yourself with others.

The group that expressed their feelings experienced advantages relative to the other group in every category including self-awareness, comfort around others, and contentment. The group that refrained from sharing their feelings not only was less assertive but tended to feel less confident and more awkward around others and to be less successful in accomplishing goals. The group's greater need for social approval might explain this finding.

Consider why self-expression is such a crucial component of EQ. If you genuinely want others to like you and don't share your authentic self with them or refrain from empathizing with their situation in a compassionate way, your relationships will suffer. Your health will also suffer because you aren't getting your needs met when you favor compliance over self-care.

Self-expression is one of the means through which you can communicate and attain your goals. We will explore effective communication later in this book.

The way that you talk to yourself is another form of self-expression. It is how you silently express your innermost thoughts. Because thoughts, feelings, and behaviors are interconnected, your self-talk can determine how you feel and affect your performance. If you want to manage your emotions, you need to pay attention to your inner dialogue.

Are you harder on yourself than you are on others? Perhaps you tell yourself that you should "just get over it" after a challenging experience or that you are "a failure" because the task you worked on did not turn out as well as you had hoped. This approach lacks compassion. There is a better and more effective way to relate to yourself if you want to increase resilience and performance.

Think about somebody else who is struggling. Say your friend Sally had the same struggle that you are currently facing and she was sitting right next to you. What would you say to her? Imagine how you might try to comfort her, or how you would advise her to move forward with her situation. Then, apply some of that compassionate talk to yourself. While it might seem like being hard on yourself is the key to improvement, the opposite is true. Compassion builds you up to face challenges and stressors and is what leads to greater resilience.

If you can have compassion for others but not for yourself, tune into your inner voice. Determine whose voice is speaking to you. Does it sound like someone in your life, perhaps a family member or your boss?

To counter this harsh and judgmental voice, identify someone kind. It can be someone you know or even a fictional character. Imagine inserting this voice of compassion into your head to counteract the other very critical voice. This can help you distill the negativity, instill more compassion, and become more resilient to perform in a demanding environment.

CONCLUSION

To respond to pressures in the workplace, you must have clarity of thought, think objectively, and remain calm. Mastering your emotions is part of your arsenal for becoming effective. To begin this journey, you must first be aware of what you are feeling, allow yourself to face these emotions, and extract lessons from them.

Negative emotions stem from worried, judgmental, or other unhelpful thoughts. By applying mindfulness, you can alter your interpretations of events and gain more control over your feelings. Focusing on responding mindfully rather than reactively demonstrates a form of self-control.

Emotional mastery results from mindful habits of self-care, self-examination, and self-expression. When you know yourself, you can communicate to others what you feel in order to get your needs met.

By tackling your anxiety from various angles, you will be better prepared to manage it when it arises. This will give you the proper balance and motivation to stay focused on what matters so you can get through your day with ease and peace of mind.

CHAPTER 7

Zone of Optimal Performance

If you care about achievement, you care about your performance. The quality of your performance is affected by your arousal level. Both high and low arousal levels lead to compromised work, so it is important to understand what determines these states of arousal and how to manage them. By doing so, you will enter the zone of optimal performance (ZOOP).

When you become overly aroused, you experience high levels of anxiety. For instance, when work demands are high, you go into overdrive, trying to get tasks done at a frenetic pace. Over time, this leads you to feel drained and burned out (figure 7.1).

While it is commendable that you dive into action when faced with a challenge, paradoxically, you need to lower your arousal. By reducing activation, you can release tension and prevent exhaustion. You can accomplish this by improving your time management skills by minimizing distractions, prioritizing essential tasks, undertaking a realistic amount of work, and delegating everything else. Additionally, avoid taking on too many responsibilities. Remember, if your job requires that you do more than is feasible in the time you have, you need to put some boundaries in place.

It might be difficult to catch yourself in the moment of an elevated arousal state to implement change. If that is the case, sit down and think about past instances where you became frenetic or shut down. List what events led to this behavior, how

FIGURE 7.1   Zone of Optimal Performance (ZOOP).

they made you feel, and what you would do differently if you were to do them over again. Look for patterns of thinking, feeling, and behaving, and you will be on your way to a more mindful understanding of yourself.

The more you can see your tendencies, the more you can plan accordingly. Create a "when-then" contingency plan for how to handle commonly triggering situations. Decide in advance what you will do by stating, "When this happens, then I will . . ." For example, if you notice a pattern that when you are up against a time crunch, you turn into the "Energizer Bunny," rushing about and feeling overwhelmed, consider doing the opposite. Your plan can read, "When a deadline is stressing me out, I will sit in a quiet place and meditate on what is the most essential task that I need to get done to push the project forward, and then I will focus only on that essential item." This can help you stay grounded and centered while avoiding unnecessary stress.

On the other end of the spectrum, you might experience hypo-arousal. This is where you underperform and typically results from sticking to your comfort zone. Instead of operating frantically, trying to accomplish those to-do items, you are more likely to disengage from the work. If you find yourself procrastinating, avoiding, or feeling bored on the job, you are disconnected. Start paying attention to body signals to get out of your head. Incorporate exercise into your routine so you can handle and thereby release the physical stress that you carry around. This will help you restore your energy, improve your focus so you can become more integrated, and free you to do your best work.

One evidence-based technique that can help you overcome procrastination is temptation bundling. Research by Dr. Katherine Milkman, a professor at the Wharton School at the University of Pennsylvania, focused on how to improve self-control by limiting access to temptation.[1]

While we all know how vital it is for us to exercise, getting to the gym might be difficult. In her study, Dr. Milkman set out to discover what level of motivation would be most successful in getting 226 students and faculty members to engage in physical activity.

Milkman placed participants in three distinct groups. The first group received an iPod and was able to access audiobooks only at the gym. Members in the second group had audiobooks loaded onto their personal iPods and were encouraged to listen to them only at the gym. The third group received a gift card and encouragement to work out more.

The results showed that the first group worked out 29 percent more than the second group and 51 percent more than the third group. The relative success of the first group resulted from bundling the temptation of the audiobooks with the challenging activity of working out, which increased the group's motivation and follow-through in facing the challenge.

Consider how you might physically restrict access to temptation to boost your performance in challenging tasks. Notice that the temptation used in the study did not sabotage the results of the challenge. If you are interested in optimal performance, don't load yourself up with sugary foods as a reward. This may give you immediate energy but will only lead to your energy dropping in a short while. Instead, consider a more inspiring, motivating, or relaxing reward such as a ten-minute meditation, stretching, or a music break.

When in a hypo-aroused state, in order to release negative emotions you are more likely to do things without being aware. For some people, emotional eating becomes their retreat from stress. You might recall stuffing food into your mouth, unaware of how much you are eating until you have reached the bottom of the ice cream container. If this is happening with you, there is a solution that has nothing to do with dieting. Instead, you need to become more mindful of your emotional state and deal with it effectively.

If you find that when you feel pressed to perform, you tend to run away to social media, invade the refrigerator, or distract yourself with mindless television, take some time out to regroup. Go for a walk to clear your head. Engaging in physical movement can release pent up energy and help you get into your body. This is also a form of self-care that will restore your energy and improve your focus on the task at hand.

The goal is to function in the ZOOP. When you are in the "zone," your performance is optimal because you are practicing self-awareness and self-management. This mindfulness will also let you know when you need to incorporate self-care. When you are in the ZOOP, you are more engaged with your work because you have the appropriate energy and are prioritizing the most crucial tasks. You are stretching yourself to achieve goals outside of your comfort level, but not ones so audacious that they create panic.

TABLE 7.1 Identifying Your Coping Strategies

When you feel stressed, what is your go-to comfort?

☐ Web surfing
☐ Playing video games
☐ Watching YouTube videos
☐ Engaging with pornography
☐ Daydreaming
☐ Browsing social media
☐ Shopping on Amazon
☐ Smoking
☐ Using drugs or alcohol
☐ Eating

Which of these healthy alternatives can you substitute instead?

☐ Meditation
☐ Taking deep breaths
☐ Listening to music
☐ Walking in nature
☐ Chatting with a friend
☐ Drinking water
☐ Taking a bath
☐ Other: _____

To enter the ZOOP, start each day with the intention to accomplish what is in the best interest for you and your family. Each time you engage in an action, ask yourself if it aligns with your intention.

What helps keep you in the ZOOP is continued self-care, social support, and a positive mindset while continuing to push

---

TABLE 7.2 **Getting Into the ZOOP**

- Release tension before jumping into action and instead of procrastinating.
- Manage your time well.
- Avoid taking on too many responsibilities.
- Pay attention to body signals.
- Try temptation bundling to build healthy habits.
- Look for patterns of thinking, feeling, and behavior from past instances of hypo- and hyperarousal.
- Create a when-then contingency plan.
- Start each day with an intention that is in your best interest.
- Before engaging in an activity, ask yourself whether it aligns with your intention.
- Trust yourself to problem-solve.

---

the boundary over time. Doing difficult things and coping adaptively increase self-esteem. They change your perception of yourself, especially when you are determined to achieve your goals and don't allow initial failure to stop you short.

Resilience starts in the mind and includes a sense of realistic optimism for what lies ahead, gratitude for the goodness around you, and acceptance of anything that is not in your control or that has not gone as well as you would have liked.

True control is trusting that you can handle anything that comes your way because you know it is temporary. The key to exerting control lies in the mastery of emotions that govern your actions. Cultivating curiosity about your thoughts is essential; it dismantles the presumption of their absolute accuracy. Negative thoughts should not be permitted to sow seeds of anxiety about the future. Instead, question whether these thoughts are based in reality or not, and let your intuition guide you.

CONCLUSION

Your arousal level is a good indication of your performance. By paying attention to your behaviors, you can gain insight into whether or not you are performing in the optimal zone. Put your self-competency skills into practice to increase mindfulness and bring yourself into the ZOOP.

When you boil it down, the heart of the matter turns out to be trust. You have to be able to trust yourself to problem-solve and to know that even though you are imperfect, you can improve over time with the right intention, mindset, and actions.

By focusing on what you can control, you can regulate your emotions and behaviors and make good decisions. Know that you are capable, and with the right effort and hard work, you will build resilience and succeed.

Social Competency

Being in control of yourself is highly valuable, though it is your relationships that are the most critical aspects of your existence, as you will learn further in this book. This is why developing your social competency is vital to cultivating the best possible relationships with others and feeling connected to them.

Social competency spans three chapters. The first, which is chapter 8 of this book, focuses on empathy, a skill that helps you better understand another person's situation. Building on this understanding, you will be more adept at managing your relationships with others, which is the focus of chapter 9. In chapter 10 you will learn skills for effective communication. This is where you bring together your self-management and empathy skills to effectively navigate your relationships.

While emotional intelligence is a highly valuable skill in the workplace, few people are actually trained in this. It has been shown to lead to greater success than your rational intelligence, which makes sense. People who are relatable and empathic and who are not overly emotional or irrational make better leaders. And even if you are not in a leadership role, when you are likable and relatable, you go farther in your career.

Social Awareness   Relationship Management

Social competency.

CHAPTER 8

Empathy

In the story of Peter and the Wolf, the bird and the duck have an exchange. The bird says to the duck, "What kind of bird are you if you can't fly?" To this, the duck retorts, "What kind of bird are you if you can't swim?"[1] Each is seeing the world from their point of view, which makes it harder to relate to the other. For the two birds to truly connect, they need to look at the situation from the other's perspective. This is what we call empathy.

When an event stirs you, you can apply your self-awareness skills to recognize what you are feeling and why you are feeling it. With empathy, you are applying this process to another person's experiences. If, for instance, your manager is doing something that is upsetting you, try to put yourself in their shoes and consider: Why are they acting like this? What do I know about them and their situation that can shed light on this for me? What might be going on behind the scenes? The better you can understand what makes other people tick, the more easily you will be able to relate to them.

When someone tells you about a personal struggle, practice active and empathic listening. Resist the urge to judge the person or the situation. Avoid the temptation to interject with your own experiences or rush to propose a solution. Remember, you don't need to fix their problem. Instead, direct your focus toward grasping the "what" and "why" of their situation—what emotions they are experiencing and why those emotions have arisen.

Once you've gained a deeper insight into their emotional state, try to connect with their feelings on a personal level. Reflect on moments in your life when you've encountered similar emotions by asking yourself, "When have I felt something similar to what this person is describing?" This empathetic approach fosters a stronger, more supportive connection.

As human beings, we are wired for connection. That is why relationships and our management of them are crucial to our success. We want to feel connected. We *need* to feel connected. It is when there are interfering factors that conflicts can arise or lead us to disengage.

Psychologist Richard Ryan notes that "one of the reasons for anxiety and depression in the high attainers is that they're not having good relationships. They're busy making money and attending to themselves and that means there's less room in their lives for love and attention and caring and empathy and the things that truly count."[2]

In a 2016 survey conducted by the National Opinion Research Center at the University of Chicago, Emma Seppälä and Marissa King found a significant correlation between work exhaustion and loneliness. When you are more focused on production than connection, your work can quickly drain you and leave you feeling lonely. Conversely, when you have social support at work, burnout rates decline as work satisfaction and productivity rates rise.[3]

While social support comes in several forms, the type of support most helpful to diminish burnout is emotional support. This includes empathy, love, and understanding. When people burn out, however, they tend to want more instrumental support to help them get things done. Instrumental support is most helpful when it is coupled with emotional support. A work culture that allows you to adjust your hours so that you can better attend to family demands is indirectly providing emotional support.

Emotional support is so vital to workers' job commitment that even the perception of such support can increase engagement. It turns out that when your boss is understanding of your family demands, you are more willing to put in long hours on the job, and, despite working longer hours, you are less likely to reach burnout when you receive this workplace emotional support.[4]

In this chapter we are going to focus on how to harness empathy to understand others better and then couple that understanding with our competency skills of self-awareness and self-management to maneuver around conflict and build healthy relationships.

ARE YOU OVERLY EMPATHETIC?

Empathy is an essential skill for relationships. If you are in the helping field, chances are that instead of struggling to understand others, you may have the opposite issue. You might be so empathetic that you experience compassion fatigue.

Compassion fatigue is when you feel so much for another person that you end up feeling emotionally exhausted. This happens especially when you put in a tremendous effort to help someone else but are not seeing the desired results. Nurses are notorious for experiencing this phenomenon. The nature of their job is to meet the needs of their patients. They are drawn to their field because they are caring, but the long hours and heavy demands can lead them to a state of emotional saturation, especially when they sacrifice their own needs in the process.

An online blog for nurses, *Nurse Buff*, provides insight into how this unfolds by sharing statements from nurses who have experienced compassion fatigue. For example, a nurse from Maryland shared: "I've been working hard to take care of my critically ill patient. Sometimes, I don't even mind skipping my meals and ignoring my urge to drink or pee just to keep up with his nursing care demands. He thankfully recovered but one day he got off from his bed and fell. When I saw him sick again, I was crushed."[5]

I have discussed the importance of self-care to maintain a balanced lifestyle and recover the energy expended throughout the workday.

Compassion fatigue is a version of over-engagement that leaves you in a deficient state and more vulnerable to disappointment when your self-sacrifices do not give you your desired results.

To avoid this emotional drain, you need to shift your perspective. Consider how you can be there for somebody without taking on their distress or total responsibility for their wellness. Keep in mind the big picture idea of how your work brings a sense of purpose to your life rather than honing in on each individual you are helping and putting all your "purpose eggs" in that basket. Know that you do the best you can without over-giving to any one individual so that you can sustain your energy in the long run.

When you reach compassion fatigue and burnout, you have less capacity for empathy. As mentioned previously, one of the main signs of burnout is cynicism, which is when you lose your ability to relate to others and when you max out. This is why you should simultaneously channel your empathy for others alongside empathy for yourself.

WHEN EMPATHY IS A STRUGGLE

It might seem challenging to apply empathy during a conflict. If you feel blamed for something that is not your fault or over which you have no control, you are likely to focus your efforts on defending yourself rather than tuning in to the other person's point of view. While this is understandable, it is a reactive response, and it will only fuel the conflict more.

To de-escalate a conflict, you need first to apply your self-competency skills. Notice what feelings are coming up for you. Take a deep breath and keep those feelings under control in whatever way works best. Only then will you be able to apply this more advanced skill of empathy, which requires that you understand the other person. It does not mean that you have to agree with them.

Always keep in mind when you are interacting with others that your goal is to connect with them. When you are defensive or accusatory, you are saying, "I am separate from you," which works against your goal. Connection is an art that requires mastery over time, but if you keep this premise at the forefront, it will help you be mindful of your responses.

You might find it hard to offer apologies when appropriate because you worry about losing face. This is an indication of all-or-nothing thinking. Saying "I'm sorry" takes humility, but it makes others appreciate you more. In essence, you are acknowledging your mistakes and the other person. Try to see the situation from their perspective and consider whether you would want an apology if you were the one wronged. By offering an olive branch, you are making a statement that you value the relationship more than your ego.

You might find it challenging to apply empathy if you internalize other people's actions as an indication of how they think or feel about you. This is true whether you know the other person or not.

IMAGINE THE FOLLOWING SITUATIONS

Scenario 1: You are taking a family walk in the morning to drop your kids off at school. You want to hold your partner's hand during the stroll, but so do both of your kids. When your partner opts to hold onto your children's hands rather than yours, you decide to break off from the group because you feel shunned.

Scenario 2: You are a safe driver. You stop, look, and follow the rules. You get to a four-way intersection and it is your turn to go through, but a car crosses in front of you. You have to wait a few more seconds for that car to pass so you can finally go. You feel disrespected and annoyed.

Scenario 3: You are on vacation. Your boss contacts one of your accounts to let them know that he is changing their terms. You find out about the change when you return to the office, and you are fuming about the sabotage your boss is enacting without discussing it with you first.

In each of these situations, you can read into the other person's intentions. Or you can make it about you, which will make you feel angry at the other person and possibly badly about yourself.

When you tell yourself that what is happening is an indication that the other person does not care for or respect you, you will become upset. These interpretations result in a spiral of negative emotions, which can sometimes lead to reactivity.

NEWS FLASH: IT IS NOT ALWAYS ABOUT YOU

Think about it. People are focused on themselves more often than not. They want the fastest, biggest, and best rewards, and this blinds them to how their actions may cause harm to others.

When your partner chooses to hold your children's hands on the walk to school, it is not because he does not want to keep your hand. It is because his focus is on holding your children's hands.

TABLE 8.1   Tips for Applying a Healthy Amount of Empathy

- Practice active listening: Give your full attention, avoid interrupting, and paraphrase to ensure understanding.
- Seek to understand: Try to see the situation from the other person's perspective, even if you don't agree.
- Validate emotions: Acknowledge and validate the other person's feelings without judgment.
- Relate personally: Share a similar experience, if appropriate, to foster connection and empathy.
- Offer support: Provide emotional support and reassurance without taking on their problems.
- Self-regulate: Before responding, take a moment to calm yourself and center your emotions.
- Avoid defensiveness: Stay open-minded and receptive to feedback.
- Take responsibility: Apologize sincerely when necessary and acknowledge your role in the situation.
- Avoid assumptions: Refrain from making assumptions about others' intentions or motivations.

When that driver takes your turn at the intersection, it is because they are focused on getting to their destination quickly. You just happen to be another car on the road.

When your boss goes behind your back, it is because they want to look good and feel in control. They likely does not have an agenda against you.

The more you can zoom out and look at the big picture and try to think about what makes other people tick, the less you will personalize what is happening and be able to let things go. So stop inserting yourself into other people's brains, assuming you know why they do what they do. Stop inserting poison into your mind and filling it with ideas of bad intent. Adjust your expectations, take a deep breath, and focus on your intentions rather than those of others so you can lighten your load.

CONCLUSION

Empathy is a skill that helps you create human connections. It requires that you take into consideration the other person's experience so you can better understand them. Ultimately, this understanding leads to important protection against burnout: social support. Though it is important to keep your support of others in check, too much or too little can bring you out of balance.

CHAPTER 9

Relationship Management

While empathy builds a bridge between yourself and others, what can help direct your interactions is an understanding of communication styles.

There are four styles of communication: passive, aggressive, passive-aggressive, and assertive. These styles are driven by our underlying beliefs concerning the significance of our own needs compared to the needs of others.

Let's illustrate this with a common scenario: Imagine your boss requests you to stay late to complete a project, even though you already have evening plans. Your choice of communication style in this situation reflects your belief system.

Passive style: If you tend to be passive, you prioritize your boss's needs over your own, believing your needs to be of lesser importance. Consequently, you might sacrifice your evening plans and stay late at the office. However, this approach can lead to resentment over time and even result in sporadic bursts of aggression as your frustrations accumulate.

Aggressive style: On the other hand, an aggressive communication style signifies that you consider your needs more important than others'. In this case, you may simply say "no" to your boss without considering the circumstances. While this might safeguard your own needs, it can damage relationships and create an impression of selfishness.

Passive-aggressive style: The passive-aggressive style combines elements of both passive and aggressive communication. It is rooted in the belief that "my needs are more important than yours," but it aims to avoid direct conflict. Instead of outright denying their boss's request, a passive-aggressive person might reluctantly agree but then fail to follow through on their promise. This style, though it may temporarily sidestep confrontation, often results in negative consequences when the truth emerges.

Assertive style: The assertive communication style represents a balanced belief that both your needs and those of others hold importance. It embodies self-awareness, empathy, and a willingness to engage in negotiation, making it a more constructive and effective approach to communication.

Understanding these communication styles can greatly influence the quality of your interactions and help you navigate various situations with greater success and harmony.

ADAPTING COMMUNICATION STYLES FOR EFFECTIVE INTERACTION

Paying attention to how others communicate tells you about their beliefs and can help guide your interactions with them. For passive people, it is best to appreciate them and then elicit from them what they need. Encourage them to advocate for themselves and show them that they are safe to do so with you.

For aggressive people, use reflective statements such as "I can see how important this is to you. I wonder if we can find a solution that meets both of our needs." This helps them feel seen by you and will make them more likely to take your needs into account.

If someone is passive-aggressive, you might let them know that you don't judge them for wanting to get their needs met and that they can feel free to share them with you instead of just telling you what you want to hear. Let them know you prefer their authenticity over their compliance.

Because assertive people are already considering both sides, they are easiest to negotiate with in an effective way. Chances are you will not need to manage their communication too much.

ASSERTIVE COMMUNICATION

Marsha Linehan, the founder of Dialectical Behavioral Therapy (DBT), came up with an acronym that can serve as a guide for asserting yourself. It is a seven-step solution called DEAR MAN.[1]

The first four steps describe *what* to say and the order in which to say it:

Describe the facts. When you disagree with someone, you want to get them on the same page as you by stating the facts. For example, you might state to your boss, "Over the past month, I have stayed late at work six different times to meet deadlines." By objectively describing the situation, you are more likely to get them to agree, an indication that you are seeing eye to eye.

Express your feelings. Now that you have described the scenario factually, you have an opportunity to talk about how you feel about it. Continuing with our former example, what you might say to your boss is: "I understand that we are in a crunch period and I want to be a team player, but this cuts into my time with my family and does not allow me as much of an opportunity to recover from the stress of the day." By using "I" statements, you reduce any possible friction.

Assert Your Needs. This is where you make a direct request for things to change. Sticking to our example, you might add,

"I would like to minimize these late nights to no more than once a week."

Reinforce Your Request. Keep in mind that people often find change difficult. Whenever you are asking to change the status quo, expect to be met with resistance. In this step, you are motivating the change. This can take two different forms. The first is positive reinforcement, where you explain the benefits. For example, you might say, "Having proper rest would allow me to come in fully restored the next morning so I can bring my best self to work."

In *Influence*, Robert Cialdini explains that when you give someone a reason for what you are doing, you are more likely to get them to comply with you.[2] So, when you explain why you need to cut out at five o'clock, it will be better received than if you just state your wish with no explanation.

Alternatively, some situations may call for negative reinforcement in which you explain the consequences of not changing a behavior. If, for instance, your boss has an aggressive communication style and shows a lack of empathy for your needs, you might say, "If I continue to stay late night after night, I will surely burn out, and I won't be as capable of doing my work well."

Hopefully, whatever conflict you are facing does not require such dire measures as threatening to leave your job if things don't change, but it might. If the situation goes against every grain of your being, you must listen to your intuition. Otherwise, you will become disempowered.

Now that you know what to say, we will examine the second half of the process, which reveals *how* to practice assertiveness:

Mindfulness. You need to stick to your agenda regardless of what fears or thoughts might come up that attempt to cloud your mind or what tactics the other person tries to throw out to distract you. If your boss talks over you, attempts to change the subject, or becomes defensive, you can either ignore them and continue on or become a broken record. You might start from the top until they gets the message that you mean business. You might even shift gears and use the DEAR part to address what is happening between the two of you in that moment. It might sound something like:

- "I noticed that as I'm explaining something that's important to me, you keep interrupting [describe]."
- "This is upsetting because it seems like you don't want to listen to what I have to say [express]."
- "I would appreciate it if you could give me two minutes to explain myself through [assert]."
- "That would mean a lot to our relationship [reinforce]."

Appear Confident. This is imperative if you want to be taken seriously. Be aware of your body language, tone of voice, and filler words. If you have an in-person conversation, make sure that your posture is erect, that you make eye contact, and that you speak up so the other person can hear you. Keep an open stance. Closed stances (e.g., crossing your arms) may signal defensiveness. If you are really in tune with the other person, you might find that you mirror their position. Remember, you have an effect on others, and by staying aware of your body, you can come across as more inviting. Paying attention to the other person's body language can also reveal unspoken truths and can help you with complex reflections (see chapter 10). Lastly, pay attention to what you are saying. You want to sound like you are serious about your request. Avoid using phrases such as "I

TABLE 9.1 **Learning to Assert Yourself**

The table below identifies communication styles of a person with whom you are interacting and indicates how to approach them assertively.

Communication Style	Assertive Approach
Passive	• Appreciate them. • Elicit their needs. • Encourage them to advocate for themselves. • Help them feel safe with you.
Aggressive	• Use reflective "I" statements that express how you understand them. • Be curious about finding a solution that fits both of your needs.
Passive-aggressive	• Let them know you don't judge them for getting their needs met. • Encourage them to be transparent rather than telling you what they think you want to hear.

---

think" or "I don't know." These indicate that you are feeling intimidated or unsure of yourself. When you take yourself seriously, others are more likely to take you seriously, as well.

Negotiate a win-win situation. By now you have asserted your request, but remember: If you believe that the other person's needs are also important, it is time to bring the conversation back around to them. This is where you check back in with the other person and see how your request fits in with their needs.

When conflict arises, if you can look at the situation from different angles and focus on the solution rather than assigning blame, you will have an easier time reaching a resolution and keeping your professional relationships intact.

CONCLUSION

By looking at communication through a lens of needs, you can gain great insight into what people believe and why they behave as they do. You can then customize your approach to their style. Through assertive communication, you can minimize conflict and get both your needs and those of the other person met.

CHAPTER 10

The Essentials of Effective Communication

When you talk, you are only repeating what you know.
But if you listen, you may learn something new.
THE DALAI LAMA

Think about a time when you had a strong urge to share an experience with someone else. Perhaps, during times of trouble, you wanted the other person's support or understanding. If you experienced a conflict with someone in your life, you might have felt tempted to communicate to them why what they are doing is problematic. This is your opportunity to assert yourself.

When you are in conversation with someone, you want to feel heard, understood, and validated. The other person may not necessarily agree with your position, but if they are respectful and listen carefully, and if you think they "get you," that alone will meet some of your needs.

Now that you are able to tune into what you would like when you are sharing something difficult with another person, let us flip the script. It is time for you to be on the receiving end and to do so effectively.

STEP 1: REFLECTIVE LISTENING

Very few of us have ever had training in how to listen. Many of us are born with the ability to hear, but listening is an art.

Imagine you are arguing with your coworker, roommate, or romantic partner. You may be so worked up that all you want to do is jump in and tell your side of the story. There might be a part of you determined to convince the other person why they are wrong and you are right. This impulse is natural. But being "natural" and "effective" are two different things.

To have quality relationships, you need to contain yourself even in the heat of the moment. You will have a chance to give your version of the story, but it's critical you first listen intently to the other person. When you listen without an agenda because you want to truly understand what the other person is feeling, thinking, and wanting, you have information you can later leverage in problem-solving.

Let's take a deep dive into what quality listening means:

- You agree to understand the other person before you tell them what you have to say.

- You reflect to them what they said.

- You see whether they agree with your summary statement. This is an invitation for them to add anything you may have missed. You can then re-summarize to ensure you got everything right this time.

- Only after they feel understood do you share what is on your mind.

This process provides role modeling. If the other person is not trained in listening the way you are, you can remind them of how you took the time to understand them and that you would like them to do the same for you. Ask them to check in with you without jumping in to make their point.

STEP 2: EMPATHIC UNDERSTANDING

To be truly effective, you are not just listening for content. You want to read between the lines, carefully examine body language, and find out what the person is feeling. By understanding the other person's emotional position, you can put yourself in their shoes and try to sense what it must be like for them. This does not mean that you have to feel their pain and overexert yourself emotionally. You can just relate to their experience as an emotional being.

Reflections are used in Motivational Interviewing (MI), a form of therapy that focuses on helping people resolve their ambivalence and overcome their resistance by mirroring their experience back to them.[1] According to MI, there are two kinds of reflections: (1) simple reflections, which focus on the content of what the person is saying, as in paraphrasing, and (2) complex reflections, which focus on the emotions and meanings behind what is said. To be able to reflect in such a way requires deep listening. It may require you to jump ahead and fill in the blank when the other person has not yet said what they mean. According to William Miller, the co-creator of MI, "Two-thirds of the change in therapy clients is attributed to accurate empathy."[2] The same outcomes are expected outside of a therapeutic setting. Empathy can help you effectively understand the other person in order to find a fitting solution to the problem.

Empathy is not the only helpful tool in understanding others. There is also the use of compassion, where you show caring and a willingness to help. According to the Dalai Lama, compassion is an uncompromising attitude that remains constant regardless of the other person's actions. It is a commitment to stay kind and focus on removing the other person's suffering no matter what they do. While the Dalai Lama acknowledges that this is a challenging practice, he advises that you start by removing anger and hatred from your heart.[3]

STEP 3: SHARING YOUR POINT OF VIEW

Now it's your turn to engage in the conversation. You've demonstrated patience by first seeking to understand the other person's perspective. To maintain effective communication, it's crucial to express yourself in a manner that the other person can truly hear and comprehend. Achieving this requires you to steer clear of blame or criticism, as these often trigger defensiveness in the other party.

Instead, adhere to these guidelines:

1. *Stick to the facts*: Begin by sharing the objective events that have transpired. For instance, if a colleague consistently arrives late to meetings, you might say, "I've noticed that in the past three team meetings, you've arrived 15 minutes after the scheduled start time."

2. *Find common ground*: After presenting the facts, initiate the conversation by highlighting elements that the other person is likely to agree with. In the

case of the late-arriving colleague, you could add, "I understand that everyone's schedule can be hectic, and unexpected delays happen to all of us from time to time."

3. *Express your emotions with "I" statements*: Following their agreement on the objective facts, share your emotions in response to the situation. Instead of attributing your feelings directly to their behavior, use "I" statements to focus on your emotions. For instance, you might say, "When these delays occur, I feel frustrated and find it challenging to keep the meetings on track."

4. *Ensure understanding*: Gauge their understanding and empathy for your feelings. It's important that they grasp your emotional perspective. For instance, you might ask, "Can you understand how these delays might affect the flow of our meetings and how I feel about it?"

5. *Proceed to your point of view*: Once you are satisfied that they comprehend your emotions and perspective, it's your opportunity to share your point of view or any concerns you may have. For example, you could continue, "I believe that punctuality is crucial for efficient teamwork, and I'd appreciate it if we could work together to find a solution."

By following these guidelines, you create a constructive and empathetic environment for expressing yourself and addressing issues effectively within the realm of communication.

STEP 4: EMOTIONALLY INTELLIGENT PROBLEM-SOLVING

If you have followed steps 1 and 2, you should have a good understanding of how the other person feels. By the end of step 3, they should have a sense of how you feel. Step 4 is about putting the two sides together and coming up with a solution that is satisfactory to both parties. This is not about compromising. It's about an attempt to get both people's needs met. It requires creativity, patience, and goodwill.

When the person you are speaking with feels understood, they are more open to moving the focus from the problem to the solution.

It's best to take the "teach a man to fish" approach to empowering them to solve their problem rather than trying to fix it for them. Elicit this problem-solving mindset through questions such as, "What do you think will help in this situation?" When they come up with their answers, they are more likely to follow through. If, however, they become stumped, you can ask permission to provide a suggestion. By preempting your solution with this request, you will help the person be more receptive to hearing what you suggest.

STEP 5: FINDING THE ESSENCE

In every situation, some elements repeat themselves. You may recognize a part of the current conflict because it reminds you of the arguments you used to have with a family member. To grow as an effective communicator, boil down the problem-turned-solution and see what you can learn from this experience. This can help you circumvent future interpersonal issues.

TABLE 10.1 **Tips for Effective Communication**

- Reflective listening: Listen without interruption, reflect on what you've heard, and get to an agreement before sharing your side.
- Empathic understanding: Examine body language and cultivate compassion.
- Sharing your point of view: Use "I" statements.
- Emotionally intelligent problem-solving: Find a solution that fits both sides. Elicit the answer from the other person and ask permission before making a suggestion.

Use the knowledge you gained about how you affect others emotionally and consider what lessons might be in store for you. You can also reflect on any triggers you experienced and think what you can do the next time you are in a similar situation. By extracting the essence of the case, you are setting yourself up for more effective communication moving forward.

CONCLUSION

Social competency is the key to successful relationships. It provides you with the framework for effective communication, which includes the right balance of empathy for yourself and the other person, deep listening, and problem-solving. These are vital skills that allow you not only to talk in a way in which you can be heard, but also to understand what the other person is experiencing and to come up with a solution that incorporates both sides.

Exercise for Step 1

There are many ways you can increase your emotional intelligence, but for our purposes let's start by focusing on the most fundamental of the necessary skills to help you manage your stress at work: self-awareness. More specifically, the goal of this exercise is for you to gain clarity about your needs, even if you aren't sure what your needs are.

In the interactive table below, you have three different ways to elicit your unattended needs. The first is by homing in on your emotional state. How do you feel when you are at work, given the demands and resources available to you? If, for example, you feel overwhelmed, write "overwhelmed" in column 1 of the table. Then ask yourself, "What is the story I am telling myself that leads me to feel overwhelmed?" You might be telling yourself, "This is too much for me." Whatever the thought, put it in column 2.

If you do not have access to your emotions or thoughts, it is best to notice your behavior. What are you doing that relates to burnout? For example, if you are disengaging from your work, put down "disengaging" under the third column of the table.

Finally, ask yourself, "What do I need in order to reengage in my work?" Reflect on any needs that are not being addressed. These may include feedback on how to improve, learning to prioritize, gaining social support, minimizing distractions, connecting to purpose, taking breaks, and incorporating self-care or other needs. Write down the most essential need that, if met, could change your experience at work.

If you need more space, draw a table in a notebook and label it like the table shown here.

Emotion	Thought	Behavior	Need
Overwhelmed	*This is too much for me*	*Disengage*	*Prioritize*

Empowerment

Energy, not time, is the fundamental currency
of high performance.

Jim Loehr and Tony Schwartz, *The Power*
of Full Engagement

To change your reality, you first needed to be in touch with your-self and have the skills to negotiate relationships with others. Now that you have these emotional intelligence skills under your belt, it's time to make use of them to *empower* yourself.

Burnout is about feeling disempowered, as though you lack control over your situation. You feel inadequate to manage the demands on you and start to question your competency. As we've shown, these experiences are simply symptoms of the problem, but there is a solution.

In this section, we will focus on ways to increase personal power so that you get your needs met. As you read about the various areas related to this process, beware—it may lead to quite a transformation!

CHAPTER 11

Personal Power

Often the world presents us with challenges. Work can be demanding and feel stressful. Even with the best of intentions, you might come across obstacles such as a shortage of time, a lack of energy, or a gap in your knowledge or skill set, any of which can make moving forward seem overwhelming. Precisely when you come to this point, you need to tune into your power.

Empowerment is the process of permitting yourself to act responsibly, to take control of your life, and to use your resources to get tasks done. Even when your job feels draining, when you are empowered, you wouldn't automatically opt for the easy way out and quit. Instead, you would buckle down and face your challenges.

In a recent study, researchers found that a better indicator of cardiovascular health than running on a treadmill was whether you could do 40 pushups during a timed test.[1] If you do not regularly exercise your arm muscles, doing 40 pushups might seem nearly impossible. Instead of giving up on ever being able to accomplish this feat, if you are determined to succeed, you could break up the task. Start with five pushups and add one more each day. Over time, you will build strength, and your daily practice will help keep the momentum going.

Like a runner who trains intensely before a marathon, you have to strengthen yourself to deal with hardships. In the process of increasing your inner strength, you will experience challenges, embarrassments, and repeated failures, but these are milestones along your path to make you into a warrior. A successful person does not wake up one day to realize their strength. Being successful is something you have to develop with intention and focus. When you develop personal power, you can apply it to any situation that requires you to take action or be fierce.

People often confuse confidence with motivation. They believe they will try something when they are certain they can do it, but waiting for confidence to show up is futile. Instead, we must drive ourselves by tapping into our inner strength to tackle challenges. From this perspective, confidence will result. We feel stronger knowing that we have climbed a steep mountain, that we have successfully faced a confrontation with a coworker even when we are uncomfortable with conflict, and that we persisted when giving up was an option.

The process of building confidence through facing challenges is a universal experience. However, during challenging times, when we're confronted with difficulties or setbacks, it's possible to slip into what's known as a victim mentality. This mentality often brings a sense of helplessness, and we may find ourselves feeling sorry about our circumstances and seeking empathy from others to counteract the negativity we're going through.

Accompanying this victim mindset, we tend to adopt negative thinking patterns. For instance, we might generalize excessively, believing that everyone is against us simply because one person has harmed us. This can lead us to view the world in overly simplistic terms, categorizing it as either entirely "good" or "bad."

In this state, we may not fully recognize the knowledge and capabilities we already possess. Doubts can creep in, making us question our abilities to do things we're actually capable of. It may even make us feel as if we have no choices left, leaving us with a sense of being trapped.

Although a victim mentality may help us suppress our anger, get attention and compassion from others, and bring about some momentary relief, it promotes a feeling of helplessness. It can trigger fears and anxieties and can bring about feelings of shame, guilt, and despair.

In contrast to a feeling of powerlessness or a perception of deficits, empowerment is focused on personal strengths. When you feel empowered, you can create the changes you want in your life rather than succumbing to a victim mentality. This concept emphasizes self-sufficiency, which may require you to learn new skills along the way. It requires that you take responsibility for yourself, take proactive action toward achieving your goals, and forgive yourself for any past doings.

In the song "Solsbury Hill," Peter Gabriel wrote about a spiritual experience he had when he left the band Genesis and started a solo career. In his words, "It's about being prepared to lose what you have for what you might get. . . . It's about letting go."[2]

Imagine you have a beat-up car in your one-car garage. You want a brand-new car, but so long as you hold onto the old one, you will not have room for the vehicle you desire. You can attain personal power when you let go of your story, the narrative that limits you. By letting go of the old, you make room for new opportunities to show up. Let go of your limiting ways of thinking about things, of your attachments, and of your habitual patterns so you can see the possibilities that await and make good choices through the new lens.

Energy management can sometimes lead to a paradoxical outcome. When exhaustion creeps in, our go-to activities often involve the least amount of effort, like binge-watching TV shows. It's like our brain says, "Hey, let's procrastinate!" You might even start with noble intentions, like improving your leadership skills by watching a YouTube video on the subject. But you have to remember to intentionally turn away from the video once it's done and put your newfound knowledge into action. Otherwise, before you know it, you're knee-deep into tutorials on how to fix a dishwasher you don't even own!

Whether you are losing power from activities that cause laziness or from people around you who are critical or create conflict, replace them with more positive influences that allow you to gain power.

You might find that you feel drained, that your attention is weak, or that you lack enthusiasm about most things in life. By understanding what drains your energy and closing the door to those influences, you can reclaim your personal power and find that you have the energy you need to be productive.

We will keep coming back to the topic of energy, as it is relevant to burnout's primary symptom of exhaustion and its

---

TABLE 11.1 Tips for Empowering Yourself

- With intention and focus, work to build up your inner strength.
- Persist during hardships rather than wait to feel confident before tackling difficult situations.
- Forgive yourself for anything you may have done wrong.
- Increase self-sufficiency.
- Take proactive action.
- Be prepared to lose what you have for what you might get.
- Mindfully reduce activities and affiliations with anything that makes you lose power.

solution of self-care. Energy is also applicable to self-awareness, our emotions, engagement in tasks, and mental resilience.

CONCLUSION

Empowerment is your personal power that develops with intention and focus, strengthens as you overcome mounting difficulties, and helps you stay determined in the face of challenges. Empowerment is associated with a strengths-based mindset that requires you to be self-sufficient and take responsibility. Let go of the old to make space for something new, surround yourself with positive influences, and eliminate energy drains.

CHAPTER 12

Amplifying Your Personal Power

There are two primary methods to augment your power. The first is identifying what depletes your energy and then doing the opposite. The second is being intentional about times and seasons, noticing how they affect your power, and making decisions accordingly.

ENERGY DRAINS

One of the most significant contributors to your lack of power is your mind. When you have negative thoughts or fears, you are less likely to take action and more likely to be avoidant.

An easy way to understand the importance of self-talk is to examine the influences of criticisms from others. Recall a time when you had your heart set on doing something you deemed meaningful, and you told someone else about it. The other person did not share in your enthusiasm and instead criticized your idea or said you lack what it takes to be successful. Ouch! What this sort of narrative can do is discourage you from persevering. So now imagine that this negative voice is your own. If you are telling yourself everything that could go wrong, how you will embarrass yourself if you fail, how it will be too difficult or take too long, chances are you will disengage. This negative headspace short-circuits your opportunity to stretch yourself and test your limits.

When a task feels difficult or the demands of the job seem excessive, you might find yourself overthinking, predicting catastrophes, and fearing failure. This self-deprecation leads to anxiety, which is energy depleting and therefore counterproductive. If you make excuses, you are just getting in your own way.

Perfectionism is another energy drain. It is an attitude of servitude because you are a slave to external circumstances. No matter how much you accomplish and how hard you try, it is never enough. It always feels like something is missing, like your outcomes are insufficient, and like there is a lot left to be desired.

If you are a perfectionist, you might believe that your needs come last, so you spend all your energy taking care of other people's requests. When you are overloaded, you will not ask for help. You will not delegate tasks to others because you hold firm to the idea that you "should" do it all yourself. You also lose power when you focus externally on the need for control or seek the approval of others.

Perhaps you are not quite a perfectionist, but you are a high achiever who has a go-go-go mentality. This need to continually produce can be incredibly draining. In this case, you may be focused not on quality but simply on the quantity of what you do. Not only does this approach use up a lot of your energy, but if you are working through lunch or think sleep is overrated and stay up late to get more done, your productivity will end up suffering in the end.

When it is time to recharge, you might inadvertently choose activities that zap your energy. When you are tired, if you are habitually choosing to watch television, play video games, or surf the internet because they are sedentary activities, you are not getting adequate rest. There is nothing wrong with kicking your feet up and engaging in entertainment, but these activities cannot be a substitute for proper relaxation. If you are exposed to brainwashing commercials or get caught up in comparing yourself to friends on social media, these activities will further drain you.

When your energy is low, you might be tempted to reach for something that will give you an immediate boost. While this may increase your energy in the moment, it can be problematic in the long term. If you find yourself eating junk food, consuming caffeine or sugary snacks, smoking, or drinking alcohol, it is a sign that you are energy deprived.

Being around certain people may also be an energy drain. People who take the victim role, for instance, are likely to be full of self-pity and avoid taking responsibility for themselves. Those who have narcissistic tendencies can be manipulative and focused solely on their own needs. People who try to dominate others can be intimidating and off-putting. Those who are always in a crisis mode seem to create drama wherever they go. Judgmental folks may try to make you feel insignificant so they can feel more important in comparison. And the person who is always acting helpless might elicit your sympathy and convince you to help, but you will likely find yourself caught in a futile cycle. If the person you are around is more of a taker than a giver, if by being around them you feel more negative than positive, or if you feel exhausted merely by spending time together, you need to minimize contact with this person.[1]

To increase your personal power, you need to identify your energy drains and reverse engineer them. If you have a critical mind, move beyond thought so you can see the ultimate truth. Our thoughts cloud our vision of reality. We experience feelings associated with our interpretation of events. Our perceptions are often flawed and can mislead us.

You need to have a positive outlook. Identify thoughts that stop you from having what you want and declare that you will do whatever it takes to make your goal come to fruition. Pay close attention to the language you use. It can make a big difference in how you feel and in your productivity. By quieting the mind, you can attain greater clarity, which will allow you to make decisions with greater ease and avoid potential obstacles.

Engaging in selfless acts demonstrates that you are acting out of your best interests. If, for instance, you feel stressed and frustrated about all you have to do, such as taking care of your children, keeping your home organized, and providing financially for your family, you might notice how depleting this feels. But once you redefine your actions as selfless, you stop anticipating reciprocity and drop expectations. This simple mind shift can give you more energy and help you feel empowered, knowing that you are responsible, caring, and strong.

Rather than focus on controlling your circumstances, turn inward to gain ultimate control of your mind, the intensity of your emotions, and your reactions. If you live with integrity, you can validate yourself rather than feel a need for someone else to recognize you. This can boost your confidence and help you show up charismatically.

Have compassion for yourself and slow down. Instead of focusing on getting an exponential amount of work done, focus on quality. Pace yourself and stay attuned to your energy levels throughout.

Consider what will truly replenish your energy. Sitting still and breathing can energize your body, release internal stress, and free the mind from negative chatter. Nourish your body with high-energy foods. Hydrate with lots of water. Declutter your environment and then your mind will also feel less cluttered, and you will regain your focus and vitality. Surround

TABLE 12.1 **Reversing Energy Drains**

Identify your energy drains and write below each one what you will focus on instead:

☐ Negative thinking

_____

☐ Fear of failure

_____

☐ Making excuses

_____

☐ Perfectionism

_____

☐ Not asking for help

_____

☐ Not delegating tasks

_____

☐ Having a relentless go-go-go mentality

_____

☐ Needing approval from others

_____

☐ Not getting adequate sleep

_____

☐ Not taking breaks

_____

☐ Consuming negative media

_____

☐ Eating poorly

_____

☐ Drinking alcohol

_____

☐ Smoking

_____

☐ Having a cluttered environment

_____

☐ Engaging with negative people

_____

☐ Other

_____

yourself with people who are enthusiastic, supportive, and loving.

Showing up powerfully requires you to be aware of your energy. It's like a light switch: You have to know which direction turns you on and which shuts you down. When inspecting your circumstances, consider what gives you personal power and what takes your power away. This awareness can help you make better decisions that are aligned with your integrity, your goals, and your values.

TIMES OF POWER

Energy is all around you and is continuously shifting. It changes from situation to situation, from morning to night, and from season to season. Notice how differently you feel when you wake up than when you go to sleep. If you are a morning person, you likely feel energized early in the day and sleepy in the evening. Alternatively, if you are a night owl, it might be hard to find the energy to leave your bed when the alarm goes off in the morning. It's harder still to go to bed because this is when you feel most alive and energized and have your clearest thoughts and most productive hours late into the night.

Each season brings different energy with it as well. In wintertime we feel more sluggish. There is less sunlight, and we are more likely to hunker down in the cold weather and feel the need to be still. Spring is a new beginning, and we feel revitalized to clean and organize our home. The summer can be a time of robust activity, as we have the most energy this time of year. Like the leaves of a tree, during the fall season we are ready to let go of anything that may be limiting us or draining our energy. As the seasons change, our energy can speed up, slow down, or bring us into balance.

Do you have a time of year when you typically feel burned out? One lawyer I spoke with stated that he finds himself getting burned out around the end of the year. November, December, and January are the months when he starts to feel the accumulation of stress from the year's entirety. What about you?

It is essential to understand how your energy changes with the seasons and not take a one-season approach all year. If, for example, you push yourself all year, as you might do in summer when your energy is highest, you will feel exhausted. To set yourself up for longevity, you need to tailor your approach based on the time of year.

In between each season there is a two-week period of transition. In the middle of each season change is either a solstice

---

TABLE 12.2 Times of Power Intention

Create an intention related to each of the following:

- Time of the day
  - Early bird: Focus on getting the most important and challenging tasks done early in the day.
  - Night owl: Carve out undisturbed time at night to get your work done.
- Season of the year
  - Winter: Focus on recharging through meditation, journaling, grounding, and resting.
  - Spring: Clean and organize your environment while planting seeds for new projects.
  - Summer: Combine diligent work with taking breaks, limiting distractions, and reaping what you've sown.
  - Fall: Review where you are and let go of anything that stands in the way of your growth.
- Time of transition
  - Solstice: Release the old, reflect, and journal on your findings.
  - Equinox: Cultivate inner balance through meditation and apply balance in your life through your actions (i.e., achieve financial balance).

---

or an equinox. During the summer and winter solstices the sun is farthest away from the equator, and thus we have the longest and shortest amount of sunlight, respectively. This is a time to think about what in your life you want to change. What do you want more of, and what do you want less of? During the spring and fall equinoxes the sun is closest to the equator, so we have equally long days and nights. The equinox is when there is balance in the universe, which is why it is an excellent opportunity for you to focus on cultivating more inner stability.

Listen to your body, pay attention to your energy gauge, and work in harmony with your circadian rhythm as well as with the seasons.

Be aware of what gives you power and what takes your power away. These are critical aspects of empowerment, which can alter stressful situations and provide you with the energy, confidence, and motivation to act. However, merely having power is not enough.

You need to have a developed sense of self to know what to go after and investigate the internal challenges that arise. By having clarity and removing obstacles in your path, you can mobilize your energy to continue expressing and gaining personal power.

CONCLUSION

To increase your personal power you need to eliminate energy drains (e.g., negative thinking, perfectionism, putting your needs on hold, controlling others, seeking outside approval, doing too much and recovering too little, seeking immediate gratification) and do the opposite. To this end you need to have an awareness of your energy level and employ a positive outlook, be selfless, engage in healthy and energy replenishing activities, and surround yourself with positive influences. Also, pay attention to times of the day and the season so you can be aware of when you feel most energized and in harmony with the forces around you.

CHAPTER 13

Becoming More Yourself

When you face difficult circumstances, such as exceedingly high demands from your job, it is not uncommon to experience a range of reactions to it. While some people complain because they are upset, others become anxious and easily overwhelmed, while still others take charge and become more focused. We can link the differences in these reactions to different beliefs within each person, beliefs that define how they see themselves. But what leads to these different beliefs in the first place?

Psychiatrist Murray Bowen came up with a theory about the influence family systems have on how individuated a person becomes.[1] The less your sense of self is developed, the more others will be able to influence you. If you depend heavily on external approval and acceptance, you will be more likely to adjust your way of thinking and your behaviors to please others. Alternatively, you may try to control others by telling them what they should be like and pressure them to change.

When your sense of self is well developed, you do a dance between your sense of autonomy and your reliance on others. This means that when those you are closest to become critical or rejecting, you do not allow their actions to cloud your judgment. You stay focused on your goals while acknowledging that your progress may not be accepted or understood by some people in your inner circle.

Based on this theory, it is probable that you would want to be in the latter scenario, where you feel confident and can stand your ground regardless of what feedback you receive from others. This would enable you to feel connected and avoid becoming overly dependent or easily manipulated by others.

Bowen stresses that people do not usually shift their level of self-differentiation unless they consciously make an effort to do so. If you are searching for ways to function more optimally, focus on ways to more authentically be yourself.

To become self-differentiated, you first need to understand the layout of this concept and figure out where you fall within it. To begin, think of a time when you had to make a major decision that did not sit well with your family. Perhaps you wanted to marry someone your parents did not approve of or enter a field of study that was different from the family business. Whatever the situation, reflect on your consequent behaviors. Did you listen to your inner voice, or did you capitulate under pressure? If you rebelled against your parents, did you feel guilty, or were you able to balance your decision and emotional reaction to it?

Self-differentiation consists of two elements (figure 13.1). The first is being able to tell the difference between your thoughts and your feelings. You may feel guilty about not listening to your parents, but if you have a strong sense of self you will understand where those feelings are coming from and choose your own direction. Part two of this process is choosing whether you let your intellect or your emotions guide your decision-making. The more differentiated you are, the more you let your mind be your guide.

This is a simplified understanding of differentiation. As mentioned above, there is an intricate dance you have to do between autonomy and intimacy. Being extreme in either direction can lead to problems. When you are too autonomous, you become isolated. This can lead to loneliness and depression. On the flip

FIGURE 13.1 Self-differentiation.

side, when you are too fused with others, you are not living your life the way you want to, which can create a sense of meaninglessness and propel constant anxiety about what others think of you. The latter is also a way of giving up your personal power.

To help you increase your sense of self, let us focus on seven concrete areas: responsibility, authenticity, resilience, vulnerability, self-governance, courage, and mindfulness. Wherever you may find yourself at the moment, remember that self-awareness is the first step. By recognizing where you lie on the spectrum between autonomy and connection, you can start to make the necessary changes to bring you into balance.

RESPONSIBILITY

Do you take responsibility for yourself, including for how you think, feel, and act? Or do you expect others to make you feel good? When people make comments similar to "I will be happy when . . . ," they are externalizing the responsibility for themselves. Such comments set an expectation that circumstances will change their life and create a passive stance. Focus instead on what you can do to change your life for the better so you can find the happiness you desire. This may sound something like "I am actively working on ways to improve my level of satisfaction" or "I take responsibility for my state of mind."

It is all too common to hear people say phrases like "You made me so mad!" Other people cannot make you feel anything. Your reaction to your environment or other people is your own. It is not what your environment or other people are doing that is causing your feelings. It is your interpretation and your ability to control your thoughts that lead you to feel a certain way.

The other aspect of responsibility to consider affects your beliefs about being of service to others. Do you take responsibility for "fixing" those around you who are suffering, or do you recognize that it is their responsibility to fix themselves? Remember that just like you, others need to be responsible for meeting their own needs. When you take their responsibility to do so onto yourself, you enable the person to stay stuck, which ironically is the opposite of what you want for them.

Differentiation is a balancing act, so while you are focused on becoming responsible for yourself, you are also focusing on cultivating closeness to those you care about. Be accountable to others, not responsible for them.

AUTHENTICITY

As mentioned earlier, those around you may disapprove of your plans. Being differentiated means that you stay true to yourself and continually work toward achieving your goals while letting others around you know who you are. This requires you to be clear about your identity, a process of self-awareness that results from exploring your values, needs, and desires. You are born to be unique, and it is your gift to yourself and the world when you express your authentic self.

Let's assume that you are determined to travel the world for a year. You have saved up your money, purchased your airline tickets, and are finally sharing your idea with your coworkers as you give your notice. Not everyone will be enthusiastic about your plans. When you are in a situation where the people around you are not supportive, you have a choice. You can either try to fit in and give up on your dreams, or you can stick to your plans and look to build a community of like-minded individuals. So if your coworkers criticize your plan, tap into your personal power to not let them dissuade you or bring up self-doubt. Likely, when you are traveling around the globe, you will meet others who have a similar sense of adventure to your own.

RESILIENCE

When there is interpersonal tension, your instinct might be to flee. But avoiding conflict does not solve anything and can keep you stuck in a perpetual pattern. You can focus on reducing friction by removing blame and acknowledging the other person's point of view. Even if you do not agree with them, this simple act of listening to their perspective can lower resistance. Remember that being differentiated means being internally strong and able to withstand disagreements without being easily manipulated or elusive. Being resilient means recovering from such interpersonal clashes quickly.

Let me tell you about an incident I had with a woman with whom I was splitting a lane in the swimming pool. Because it was just the two of us in the lane, I stuck to the right side for my laps while she was on the left. At one point, though, she began swimming on a diagonal, and I accidentally made contact with her. I was surprised at her reaction. She stood up and started screaming, "You should stick to your own lane!" My immediate inclination was to explain what had happened from my point of view. However, she did not receive my perspective well. When I suggested that perhaps she was sticking out into my lane, she yelled out, "Oh! So now it's my fault!" I instantly understood that my defensive response only increased the conflict. I self-corrected, reassuring her that it was no one's fault, that I wasn't blaming her, and that I wasn't complaining.

What followed further surprised me. Instead of continuing to yell, my pool partner immediately pivoted 180 degrees and said, "You are so kind!" The next thing I knew, she was introducing herself to me with her first name. She then apologized and informed me that she has a physical condition that makes it difficult for her to swim in a straight line. Indeed, she went from blaming me to admitting fault, but only when she felt it was safe to do so. This instance solidified for me the importance of non-defensiveness regardless of whether you are at fault or wrongly accused.

You can also be resilient when the conflict does not involve you directly. Judd came to see me because his girlfriend did not get along with his parents. He felt like he was in between the two parties and that he had to choose a side. This brought up feelings of helplessness that were familiar to him from childhood, when, as an only child, he watched his parents constantly argue and yell at each other. Rather than stay passive and watch an argument unfold between his girlfriend and dad, I encouraged him to acknowledge both sides and move the conversation along. By taking charge rather than sitting at the sidelines, Judd became more empowered.

VULNERABILITY

While focusing on your goals, you may recognize areas of weakness that keep you from forging ahead. This is an opportunity for increased connection where you can elicit the help of those around you and simultaneously remain responsible for your own needs. Use effective communication to let others know what you can use help with, but stay mindful not to be demanding or let your expectations get the better of you. If the person you approach is unable or unwilling to help at this time, don't ruminate or give up. Focus on people you can reach out to who are available and eager to assist you. Keep in mind that there will be needs that may not be met, so stay realistic to avoid disappointment.

Being vulnerable does not mean that you are weak. It takes courage to admit you have a deficit or that you are not perfect. It's hard to be vulnerable if you worry too much about what others will think of you. Remember, being self-differentiated and powerful means thinking for yourself. Don't let your imagination about what other people might say turn you around. The truth is, many of these projections are unfounded and usually don't happen the way you may anticipate. When someone is not on your side, you can harness your resilience to sustain your vulnerability.

SELF-GOVERNANCE

When your emotions get the better of you, they are in control and can lead you to be reactive and make poor decisions. Reflect on past instances where you were either unaware of your feelings or were overwhelmed by them. Recognize that it's perfectly normal for you to have emotional responses to events around you and that the feelings that emerge are there for a reason. Slow down enough to consider what you are feeling and why you are feeling this way. This will give you a better understanding of yourself, which you can use to make decisions that align with your goals for connection and that will not detract from your sense of self.

So often I hear from my clients that they are not even aware of their feelings; they push their feelings down so they can keep forging ahead. It is true that just because you are sad, scared, or upset, the world does not stop. You still have the same level of responsibility at your job and often at home, and having all of these feelings inside will get the better of you if you do not deal with them. Over time, their intensity increases until you feel overwhelmed by your emotions or until they manifest as disease in your body, keeping you from being able to function.

One of my clients compared her tendency to push her feelings down to pushing a balloon under water. The balloon does not stay down for long, and eventually it pops up with a vengeance. When she is going through difficult times that lead to strong negative emotions, she tends to busy herself as a distraction. She worries that facing her negative emotions will incapacitate her, and then she will be unable to do what she needs to get done.

Through our work together, she recognized that just because she was not focusing on her emotions did not mean they were not negatively affecting her. Instead of continuing to evade her feelings, she came up with a system to manage her feelings and be able to make decisions under less-than-ideal conditions. She asked herself, "What would a CEO do?" This mindset allowed her step into a position of leadership and confidence. As we practiced embracing and honoring her feelings, her distress went down. She found it helpful to acknowledge what was inside of her and put into practice what she imagined a CEO would do. This provided her with the inner guidance she needed when she was under duress.

COURAGE

We all have fears that can keep us from making progress. Even with the best intentions in mind, we can become stuck in a rut. Work to overcome your fears by focusing on your life's purpose. Steer clear of extreme thinking that leads to extreme behavior. Life is not black or white. Let the many colors of the rainbow expand your thinking. The more you understand that your brain is trying to keep you alive, the more you will be able to remind yourself that you are not in a life-or-death situation that warrants such fear. Take it one step at a time in the direction of whatever scares you. When you get to the other side, you will feel a sense of pride and increased confidence in your ability to take on other fears and challenges. This will also remove any notion that you need others to save you from your struggle or any need to use others to attain your goals.

Many of my clients have felt stuck because they lacked clarity about what they wanted. When no other options seemed viable, they just stayed stuck in their current situation and felt hopeless that it would change. It takes courage to admit that you want to change because change can be scary. It takes further courage to act in a way that brings about change. Get clear on what you want, and ask yourself what you need to do about it. Sometimes change means altering your circumstances, while other times change is simply a shift in perspective that can make all the difference.

MINDFULNESS

Your early life circumstances, especially those events that left a wound, can be triggers for future reactions. You might find that you are having strong reactions to situations that are seemingly mild. This is an invitation to work on neutralizing your triggers, a process you can engage in with a trauma-trained therapist. Regardless of whether or not you get this kind of help, remember that you need to remain present. What is happening right now has nothing to do with your past. By differentiating between the past and the present, you will be able to stay focused on the moment and enjoy it for all that it is worth. Similarly, you want to stay in the here and now rather than focus on the future. When you feel anxious or preoccupied, it is a sign that you are future-focused. One method to bring yourself back to the present moment is to ground your body by exhaling all your air several times.

Much of the process of differentiation is understanding that you have a right to be unique while focusing on creating strong relationships with others. This balancing act requires boundaries, which start in your mind. By getting clear on how you define yourself, you can establish limits about what is appropriate and what is not. You can start to differentiate between what feelings you have that are your own and those that you may have absorbed that belong to someone else. Once you identify that you are holding onto unnecessary angst, let it go.

In this sense, what is true and right for you may not be true and right for others. Release any judgments or criticisms you have about others who are pursuing their path. Replace such negative opinions with compassion and give them the same opportunities for personal growth, even when they are struggling, without either trying to deter them or save them. We all have to experience failure to learn how to improve. Accepting others for their differences and celebrating those differences will enrich your relationships.

Having a greater sense of self allows you to have the best of both worlds. You can live your life more fully, finding a sense of fulfillment from being authentic to yourself while cultivating connections with others around you. The more self-differentiated you are, the more capable you are of functioning well under stressful conditions and therefore problem-solving with increased effectiveness.

You benefit in many ways as you become self-aware and can manage your feelings. You gain more control of important life decisions, your health, and reactivity to stress or others' emotions. You establish more definitive boundaries and are less likely to engage in behaviors that do not suit you. By validating yourself rather than focusing externally on approval from others, you gain more confidence.

The more differentiated you are, the better you will be able to manage work stresses such as excessive demands on your time and energy. This is due, in part, to being able to transform your beliefs, which affect your emotional outcome and your coping. Your beliefs about meeting your needs while effectively addressing conflict help you cope even in the most intense

---

TABLE 13.1   **Enhance Your Sense of Self**

- Take responsibility for how you think, feel, and act.
- Be accountable to others, not responsible for them.
- Surround yourself with like-minded individuals.
- Reduce conflict by eliminating blame and acknowledging the other person's point of view.
- Recognize personal areas of weakness and ask for help.
- Keep expectations realistic to avoid disappointment.
- Consider what you are feeling and why you are feeling it.
- Ask yourself, "What would a CEO do?" and act accordingly.
- Focus on your life's purpose and move forward one step at a time.
- Stay focused on the present moment.
- Ground your anxiety.
- Release judgments about others.
- Accept and celebrate others' differences.
- Have compassion for other people's struggles.

---

situations because you can focus on both the circumstances outside of yourself and your inner experience.

Stress is not the enemy. Other people's agendas are not your roadmap.

You need to take responsibility for getting your own needs met. Stay true to yourself by focusing on what you desire for your life. Remain mindful of your emotions so you can manage them and make good decisions. Have the courage to be vulnerable, and learn to cultivate intimacy with, rather than dependency on, others so you can remain resilient and powerful and increase your confidence.

Once you are empowered and self-differentiated, you need to know how best to utilize your power, and for this you need to have clarity about your needs.

CONCLUSION

According to the theory of self-differentiation, external events affect people differently based on their sense of self. A poorly differentiated person focuses on external approval, whereas someone with a well-developed sense of self incorporates both autonomy and reliance on others. By separating your thoughts from your feelings and knowing which of these forces leads you to make decisions, you can become empowered and strengthen your sense of self.

CHAPTER 14

Hierarchy of Needs

As mentioned in chapter 4, Abraham Maslow claimed that our needs are hierarchical and that we must meet those needs in a particular sequence.[1] Maslow identified five human needs, and in this chapter we will discuss the first four. The final need is discussed in chapter 32.

PHYSIOLOGY

Starting with our most basic physiological needs, we focus on getting shelter, food, water, and sleep. Without these vital life-sustaining elements, it is fruitless to focus on anything else.

Since you are reading this book, chances are you have secured the first level of the pyramid (see figure 4.1). You have met the most basic needs that keep you alive. Even though this is true, when you become highly stressed in your life, your sleep suffers, you start to eat poorly, and you substitute caffeine and sugary drinks for water. So rather than take this first level of needs for granted, you must continually monitor your behaviors and make the best choices for your well-being. By doing so, you are establishing a strong foundation that will lead you to your ultimate desires.

SAFETY

Once we establish our foundation, we climb up to the second tier of the pyramid. We focus on safety issues. Beyond physical safety, we want to create stability in our lives. We attain financial security through employment, entrepreneurship, and investments. While there are good reasons why we focus so intensely on this aspect, we need to be careful, as we often get stuck here.

I have worked with many smart and talented individuals who were making far more money than I ever made at their young age. And yet, it seemed that despite their economic success, they were struggling emotionally. You might be able to relate to this, especially if you have a high-demand job that requires you to sacrifice much of yourself.

You might find that you pour all of your energy into your work, yet it never feels done. You have no choice but to stay late, and, even then, sometimes you take it home with you. If this is sounding like your story, your job is taking up two of your most valuable resources in exchange for one: time and energy in exchange for money.

Many of the people I have worked with struggle with feeling like what they make is never enough. When they get a raise, they upgrade their lifestyle. They buy fancier cars and eat at more expensive restaurants, so they need more money to continue to match their expenses. Some of them think about retirement and the need to create passive income. Planning for the future is crucial, especially because so many of them are miserable at their jobs and want an exit strategy. I am certainly a proponent of planning and creating multiple streams of income, but what I see with a lot of my clients is that they get stuck around issues of safety, so much so that they never attain the next level of the pyramid. As a result, no matter how much money they make and how great their lives may seem on the outside, they are unhappy.

People often have difficulty attracting a hefty paycheck because they believe they do not deserve it. If they are making a lot of money, they may feel like they have to stretch out their work hours to justify their pay. Others have a hard time holding onto money due to beliefs that they are not good money managers. Whether you are not making what you are worth, are working so hard that your life is out of balance, or have a hard time saving your money to create financial security, you can benefit from working on your mindset.

Our money beliefs are usually tied to our personal history and tend to go back to childhood. Consider the relationship your parents had to money. Were they struggling financially? Did they fight a lot about money? You may have picked up a notion that money is scarce. Alternatively, you may associate negative ideas with cash (e.g., greed or materialism).

Lenny came to me because he was unhappy in his relationship. His partner had a change of status after selling his stock and wanted to use his windfall to travel. Lenny could not afford to travel based on what he was making at his job. And the fact that his income was low was no accident. Money was a trigger for Lenny. We uncovered that the limiting belief that had kept him making too little was that he did not believe it was possible to make more. Lenny also considered himself a spiritual person and said he did not feel good focusing on money.

Through further exploration of these historical beliefs, Lenny realized that he indeed wanted more money so he could have the financial freedom that his partner now had. That said, he still did not believe he could get it or that he deserved an increase in pay. Because he was not making as much as he wanted, he saw himself as worthless, which made it challenging to ask for more money.

To rewire his limiting belief into one more aligned with his new goal, Lenny started reciting an affirmation daily about his worth. Within three weeks, his belief in himself had tripled. He quickly set a new financial goal, updated his resume, and began job searching. Seven weeks later, he was offered a new position with a $20,000 raise.

If you have anxiety about money or anything else, chances are you do not feel secure. Work on grounding your anxiety so you can feel calm enough to take action and progress up Maslow's Human Needs Pyramid.

LOVE AND BELONGING

Level three of the hierarchy of needs is about love and belonging and your relationships with other people, including friends, family, and your romantic partner. We are social beings, and we cannot derive real meaning from life without connections with other people. In *The Top Five Regrets of the Dying*, a palliative nurse collected the regrets of her dying patients.[2] Here are some things we can learn about life not fully lived.

"I wish I'd had the courage to live a life true to myself, not the life others expected of me." Sometimes, as an attempt to be loved and to belong, we take on other people's wishes and make them our own. We forget to listen to ourselves. We get lost. We live inauthentically to please others. So while we need connections, we need to be true to our desires and, rather than fit in, which involves changing yourself to meet others' expectations, strive to belong, meaning that you're accepted for who you truly are. Consider your behaviors and the choices you make. Are they

what you truly want? Is someone living vicariously through you even though you would rather be doing something else? Be honest with yourself.

"I wish I hadn't worked so hard." It is standard in twenty-first-century America to work a minimum of 40 hours a week with only two weeks of vacation. But if you are reading this book, you are not average. You likely fall into the high-achievers camp, which means you work upward of 50 hours per week. High achievers are often those who fail to take their vacation days. It is no wonder high achievers burn out. They have so much to prove to themselves and others, and the work feels like it is never done.

When you are on your death bed and you look back at your life, will you think you focused on the wrong things? Did you pass up on opportunities because you were too busy? Did you avoid taking the easy road, even part of the time, because you had something to prove? Did you want to feel accomplished, but never felt like what you did was enough? It is time to rethink this paradigm, so you do not end up with regrets. How can you work less, relax more, and enjoy the lifestyle you are working so hard to build?

Ana came to see me because her husband was working long hours, which left her feeling lonely and confused. She was often anxious about making advanced plans, especially for long weekends, because she knew that without something in hand, her husband would run off to the office. Sure, he had a justification. He knew he could get more work done when no one was around. He had a lot of work to do because he was part of a start-up and wanted it to succeed. From this perspective, his work ethic made perfect sense. After two decades of this pattern, however, Ana started to wonder, "How much do I really matter to him if he's never around?"

Deep down, Ana knew that she did matter to her husband and that he was a high achiever with a deep desire to feel accomplished. He wanted his family to have financial security, and he took it upon himself to be the provider for them. This made it easier to choose his work over his family because it was, in a sense, a form of self-sacrifice.

Ana's husband is not alone in this paradigm. How many times do we hear of people who work around the clock, whose entire identity is wrapped up in their work, and who, as a result, do not have much time to enjoy their life outside of work? It is often when the time has run out and only in retrospect that the high achiever realizes they have missed out.

"I wish I'd had the courage to express my feelings." Relationships are about the communication of our innermost worlds, including our needs, desires, thoughts, and feelings. We all want to be seen and understood, but if we do not express ourselves, how will others know who we really are? In many cultures, talking about feelings or simply showing feelings to others is considered a sign of weakness. We learn to zip up our emotions and keep tight-lipped. Like any limiting belief, this is one we need to challenge. It is outdated. Research confirms that holding our emotions inside can cause our foundation to crumble.[3] When you refrain from expressing yourself, your emotions can turn into physical pain and even autoimmune diseases. You suffer inside, and your relationships to others will suffer on the outside.

When someone shares a story of personal hardship, how do you think of that person? Often, we consider this an act of courage. Still, we forget that showing vulnerability brings us closer to others. When it comes time for us to be vulnerable, we often shut down. We are afraid of people's judgment. It's time to end the double standard. If you want to maintain your health and cultivate relationships, you must open yourself up as well.

"I wish I had stayed in touch with my friends." Are you so caught up in your busy life that you have no time for your friends? The older we get and the more entrenched we are in our work, the more isolated we become.

Why are friendships important? According to Aristotle, the Greek philosopher and scientist, friendships serve several purposes. He said, "In poverty and other misfortunes of life, true friends are a sure refuge. The young they keep out of mischief; to the old they are a comfort and aid in their weakness; and those in the prime of life they incite to noble deeds."[4]

Tom Rath, a former Global Practice Leader at Gallup, conducted research on friendships and uncovered three key benefits of close workplace relationships:

1. Individuals who have a best friend at work are seven times more likely to be engaged in their jobs. This heightened engagement leads to greater motivation and productivity, which benefits both the individual and the organization.

2. Employees with close friends at work report significantly higher levels of job satisfaction. This positive sentiment contributes to a more enjoyable work environment and can lead to lower turnover rates.

3. Friendships in the workplace provide essential social support, which can help reduce stress and improve overall mental health. Having supportive colleagues can lead to better coping mechanisms during challenging times.[5]

Relationships can be both stressful and stress-fighting, depending on the nature of the interaction. We are affected by our proximity to others and the level of intimacy we have with them. When you surround yourself with people who are very negative, critical, or unsupportive, you tend to shut down. When, despite your innate desire for closeness, you are unable to convert this individual into being your personal fan, you may want to run the other way. Conversely, when you surround yourself with others who are loving and supportive, you flourish. Thus, it is a prominent reminder for you to actively pursue people who are positive and encouraging, as well as environments that attract like-minded individuals.

"I wish that I had let myself be happier." As you get caught up in the rat race, you often forget to slow down and enjoy the journey. You might seek happiness in the form of accumulating material possessions but find this unsatisfying. So, why not pursue more happiness? For many, it boils down to the belief that "I don't deserve it." Maybe you believe that you aren't worthy, that you are "bad," or maybe you are unaware of your true value by not realizing when you aren't doing well. Mel Robbins wrote a book about the latter in the hopes of getting us to wake up to the truth and push the boundaries to reach our true potential. In *Stop Saying You're Fine*, Robbins outlines how we are often our own worst enemy.[6] We get comfortable in our old ways, even when they keep us miserable. We fear change, so we convince ourselves that everything is "fine."

How can you push the envelope and fill your life with greater joy?

If you could have the kind of life you only dream of, what would be different? Surely, you would not be working as hard as you are, you would not be as lonely as you feel, and you would enjoy the comforts of your life more. So why not turn that dream into a reality? With the right mindset you can.

ESTEEM

Once you've established meaningful connections with others and nurtured the friendships and love relationships you desire, the next step on Maslow's hierarchy is esteem, which involves your personal power and self-perception as you present yourself to the world.

Consider how you view yourself: Do you possess the confidence to tackle new challenges? When someone recognizes your efforts or seeks your friendship, do you truly believe you deserve it? Often, even if you've rightfully earned the comforts and relationships in your life, a deep-seated belief of inadequacy can hinder your willingness to seize opportunities for personal growth.

This belief pattern that undermines self-confidence is exemplified in the story of Jillian, a 25-year-old client who faced difficulties in her first year at her job. After receiving a poor performance review, she decided to redouble her efforts, resulting in her investing more time and energy than anyone else at the company. By the end of her second year, she was celebrated at the company party as the "Most Improved" worker. However, despite her hard-earned recognition, she couldn't shake the feeling that she didn't deserve it. Her belief in her own inadequacy remained steadfast.

A similar belief pattern manifested in her romantic relationship. She had been dating the same man for five years, and when asked about their future plans, she revealed that her boyfriend wanted to wait until he had saved enough to buy a home for them. Jillian interpreted this as a personal rejection, driving her to overcompensate in an attempt to prove herself to him. Despite his praise and affirmations, she continued to blame herself for his hesitation. Only when it was pointed out that he seemed to harbor similar feelings of inadequacy did Jillian consider an alternative perspective.

In an effort to compensate for a lack of confidence, you may have adopted the "fake-it-'til-you-make-it" approach, often trembling with anxiety, fearing that someone will unveil your perceived inadequacies. If you grapple with a sense of inadequacy or suffer from impostor syndrome, it's likely that you view others as more capable and self-assured.

It's crucial to remember that while you're acutely aware of your own anxieties and limitations, your knowledge of others is typically superficial. You don't have access to their inner struggles and doubts. Rest assured that everyone, to some extent, has regrets, makes mistakes, and grapples with insecurities.

TABLE 14.1 Prioritizing Your Needs in Terms of the First Four Levels of Maslow's Hierarchy

- Physiology
  - Make good choices for your well-being, especially when under stress.
- Safety
  - Work to eliminate any limiting beliefs about financial security.
  - Live within your means.
- Love and belonging
  - Be authentic rather than focusing on pleasing others.
  - Express your feelings to increase connections to others.
  - Work to overcome your fear of change.
- Esteem
  - Stop comparing yourself to others.
  - Replace unrealistic ideals with realistic expectations.
  - Work to overcome your fear of change.

When facing stage fright, a common recommendation is to visualize the audience members as naked. Why does this technique help ease nerves? Because by imagining everyone else as vulnerable, it empowers you and provides a sense of control.

CONCLUSION

According to Maslow, your needs are hierarchical, and you should pursue them in order, starting with the basic needs.

Meeting the four human needs of physiology, safety, love and belonging, and esteem can bring a sense of contentment. Depending on where you are in the hierarchy, this will inform what you need to prioritize.

You must first have your needs met in order to do your best work. This will allow you to focus and engage in what you are doing and feel more fulfilled by it.

Exercise for Step 2

If you find yourself drowning in a sea of never-ending to-dos, and more tasks seem to pour in continuously, it is time to strategize. Get out a pen and follow these three steps:

Step 1: In the table on the next page, list all the tasks currently on your plate under the "Task List" column. Determine which of these items are tasks that only you can do given your skills, expertise, and know-how. Put a checkmark next to those items in the column labeled "Tasks Only I Can Do." Delegate the items that you did not check to someone else. Mark these by putting a checkmark next to those under the "Tasks to Delegate" column.

Step 2: Of the items on your list that you choose to keep, which of them would have the most significant impact? Put a "1" next to the first of these items in the "Priority" column and start on that one first. Then put a "2" next to the item that would have the next most significant impact. Continue to sort through your list by asking this question for the remaining items and marking them accordingly in column 1.

Step 3: Do you have control over your schedule at work, or are other people interrupting your flow and pulling you into constant meetings?

If you deem certain meetings to be essential for you to attend, focus on those. However, any meeting that you can skip and have someone else attend in your stead and report back with what you missed would give you more time to focus on your essential tasks. Determine which meetings are not the best use of your time and communicate that to your higher-ups.

By following these three steps you will prioritize your tasks, take control of your schedule, and minimize the demands of others, freeing up your time to be maximally effective.

Priority	Task List	Task Only I Can Do	Tasks to Delegate

Engagement

Now that you are emotionally in control of yourself and in your power, you can optimize engagement in your work.

Engagement is often seen as the opposite of burnout. It occurs when you have the necessary resources to effectively manage high demands, allowing you to not only meet those demands but also thrive.

As part of the solution to burnout, I discuss what both poor and optimal engagement entail. I also explore how to achieve a state of flow, identify resources that can enhance your engagement, and provide guidance on managing your time and tasks for maximum productivity.

Engagement involves expressing yourself through your work on cognitive, emotional, and physical levels. When you are optimally engaged, your productivity tends to be at its peak.

Think about a time when you were in a state of flow, when you were so immersed in what you were doing, that the time seemed to pass by much more quickly. This is what engagement is like. It is when you are simultaneously inspired and challenged. When you are engaged in such a way, you are less distracted and will get more done.

CHAPTER 15

Poor Engagement

As are many concepts in this book, engagement is found on a spectrum (figure 15.1). On one end of the engagement range is a frenetic or overly engaged state. We often see this when demands are high, control is low, and you put everything you have into doing your best work and trying to get it all done. This lofty effort strategy may work well for a short period, but over time it will take a toll, not only on your work but on your mental and physical health.

While work demands will undoubtedly contribute to your frantic behavior, there are internal demands attributed to your personality that will also be a driving force. If you are unable or unwilling to acknowledge failure, if you neglect your personal needs, or if you are prone to anxiety or irritability while also being highly ambitious with lofty goals, then you are a contender for over-engagement.

According to Christina Maslach, a researcher on the subject of burnout, when employees are overly engaged, it may be a sign that they are stressed out.[1] Consider Julio, who works intensely all day. He stares at his computer screen and tries as hard as he can to get the work done before nightfall. But the demands of his job are so high that he feels buried by his responsibilities. In an attempt to lessen his load for the following day he stays at work late, and even when he goes home he continues working into the night.

Over-engaged   Engaged-Exhausted   Disengaged

FIGURE 15.1   Poor engagement.

On the surface, we can say that Julio is highly engaged in his work. Is he a workaholic? Not necessarily—at least if what is meant by being a workaholic is that you don't want to get away from your work. Julio might just feel so overwhelmed with the amount of work he has to get done that he is not able to step away. To an outsider it may seem that Julio is obsessive. But despite his intense focus, energy, and time invested in work, Julio would love to have more personal time and feels stressed that he doesn't but instead has to work so much.

So what will happen to Julio if his situation at work does not change? Over time his energy will wane. Now imagine yourself in Julio's position. The demands of your job have not changed, but you no longer have the energy to dive in. You notice how exhausted you feel and now experience difficulties in performing tasks. You consequently start neglecting your responsibilities and feel bad about yourself or hopeless about your work. This is what Maslach refers to as "engaged-exhausted," and it is associated with feeling worn out, having a low sense of control, and low self-efficacy. In other words, you start questioning your ability to do the work.

What we know about burnout is that it is a result of chronic stress over time. On any given day, Julio can go from being overly engaged to disengaged. Disengagement is a sign of burnout when employees emotionally detach from their work. It can occur due to either chronic overwork and stress or chronic under-utilization and boredom. In Julio's case, if his exhaustion leads him to drift too far away from the demands of his job, he will ultimately become detached.

When we are disengaged, even work that at first seemed meaningful will now feel unfulfilling. The stress of the work leads us to feel irritable and impatient. In contrast, the sense of monotony and boredom from work results in a lack of personal development, which may very well lead us to contemplate changing jobs. When we burn out, we become depleted of energy, we feel exhausted, our engagement turns into cynicism, and we become ineffective.

A 2018 Gallup poll revealed a sobering statistic: nearly 70 percent of US workers were either disengaged or actively disengaged.[2] The COVID-19 pandemic, a seismic shift in the workplace, unexpectedly led to a surge in employee engagement. In mid-2020, engagement rates reached a record high of 40 percent, a significant increase from pre-pandemic levels. This uptick was likely fueled by the transition to remote work, which offered many employees improved work–life balance and flexibility.[3]

As the world gradually returned to normalcy, engagement levels began to fluctuate. In the second quarter of 2024 a slight improvement was observed, with the rate rising from an 11-year low of 30 percent to 32 percent.[4] While this represents a positive trend, it's clear that there is still significant room for

TABLE 15.1 Identifying Poor Engagement

Next to each item in in the table below, mark 1 in the "Yes" column for items that correspond with your current situation and 0 in the "No" column for those that don't. Each "Yes" answer counts as one point.

Next, count how many items from questions 1–6 (overly engaged/frenetic), 7–12 (engaged-exhausted), and 13–18 (disengaged/underchallenged) you answered "Yes" to and tally your totals under each heading. The area where you have the highest total score reveals how your engagement is poorly affected.

		Yes	No
1	Demands are high.		
2	Control is low.		
3	I am highly ambitious.		
4	I am unable or unwilling to acknowledge failure.		
5	I neglect my needs.		
6	I am prone to anxiety or irritability.		

Overly engaged/frenetic total =

		Yes	No
7	I have low energy.		
8	I find it difficult to perform my regular job duties.		
9	I have been neglecting my responsibilities.		
10	I feel bad about myself.		
11	I feel hopeless about work.		
12	I have low self-efficacy.		

Engaged-exhausted total =

13	Demands are too low.		
14	I feel detached from work.		
15	Work feels unfulfilling.		
16	I am impatient.		
17	I feel bored at work.		
18	My work lacks opportunities for personal development.		

Disengaged/underchallenged total =

improvement. Engagement levels remain below the pre-pandemic high, indicating that the workplace is not fully capturing the potential of its workforce.

The stark contrast between the potential for engagement and the reality of widespread disengagement underscores a critical issue. Clearly, the workplace is getting it wrong with such a profoundly negative impact on employees. Now that you know what makes the difference between engaged and disengaged and the difference between optimally engaged and engaged-exhausted, we'll delve deeper into the three key dimensions of optimal engagement, which I will cover in the next chapter.

CONCLUSION

When work becomes more than you can handle, you may go from being overly engaged to disengaged as you run out of steam. Despite your best efforts, as your energy depletes your work may no longer feel meaningful, and you may lose your effectiveness. Once you recognize the spectrum of engagement and your place within it, you can aim for an optimal state of engagement.

CHAPTER 16

Three Dimensions
of Optimal Engagement

Optimal engagement is work-related well-being. When you are productive without overexerting your energy resources or becoming detached, you thrive. There are three dimensions associated with engagement (figure 16.1).[1] The first is *activation*, which ranges from exhaustion to vigor. This is similar to the engagement continuum, and it also includes the physical and mental energy needed to persevere.

Research by Jari Hakanen and colleagues looked at the intersection of activation at work and the degree to which the person experienced their work to be pleasant.[2] According to this model, when workers exhibit high activation in unpleasant tasks, they experience negative emotions such as agitation, irritability, and tension, which correspond with workaholism. When, instead, they engage in unpleasant tasks with lower levels of activation, workers might feel depressed and lethargic, which corresponds with burnout.

When you focus on pleasant tasks, the outcomes you experience are positive regardless of your level of activation, but there are subtle differences. High activation on pleasant tasks leads to engagement, enthusiasm, and feelings of happiness. Low activation on these same tasks leads to feelings of contentment, relaxation, and calm.

FIGURE 16.1   The Dimensions of Engagement Model. *Source*: Schaufeli et al., "The Measurement of Engagement and Burnout."

Thus, we can conclude that it is best to focus on pleasant tasks. Your level of activation will then determine whether you have higher- or lower-intensity feelings associated with the task.

The second dimension is *identification,* which ranges from cynicism to dedication. This is about how inspired and challenged you feel by your work and your particular tasks and how proud you are of your efforts.

When activation and identification are both low, you can expect to feel exhausted and cynical. The antithesis to this, of course, is vigor and dedication, two factors which exemplify optimal engagement.

The third dimension for optimal engagement, which is not found on a spectrum, is *absorption*. This is about being so intensely and happily immersed in your work that time passes quickly, and ultimately you have difficulty detaching yourself from the task. Absorption is the opposite of the detachment (experienced by the under-challenged or the overworked) and is similar to what author Mihaly Csikszentmihalyi calls "flow."[3]

Think back to a task during which, although it demanded your full attention, your mind was clear, and focusing on it felt effortless. Because you were so immersed in the task and were

---

TABLE 16.1 Shifting Poor Engagement to Optimal Engagement

In the last chapter you identified signs of poor engagement. Now is your opportunity to turn it around.

- If you are overly engaged/frenetic or engaged-exhausted,
  - focus on changing your activation. Negative emotions such as anxiety and irritability are signs you have high activation in an unpleasant task. Exhaustion is a sign your activation level is low and the task is unpleasant.
  - focus on tasks that you find more pleasant or find ways to change your perception of the current task until it feels pleasurable.
- To increase engagement and satisfaction, focus on tasks that you enjoy where you are highly activated.
- If you are disengaged or underchallenged,
  - focus on changing your cynicism to dedication. Look for ways to become inspired.
  - find tasks that are challenging, even if they seem outside the scope of your job description.
  - consider what you want to learn in order to grow in your career.
- When you've achieved something, be proud of the effort you put in.

enjoying yourself, you were surprised to find how time flew by. That is flow.

In the next chapter we'll explore the concept of flow, a state of optimal experience where you become fully immersed in an activity. We'll discuss how to cultivate this state by setting clear goals, matching challenges to your skills, and minimizing distractions.

CONCLUSION

Optimal engagement is about activation, identification, and absorption. For the best personal experience, you need to find pleasure in your work. Engagement will then follow, and regardless of how activated you feel, if you derive pleasure, inspiration, and a sense of challenge from the task, you will experience a positive outcome. Vigor and dedication can help prevent burnout. Lastly, immersion in your work can help make it feel effortless and the time will fly by.

CHAPTER 17

Being In the Flow

The best moments usually occur when a person's body or mind
is stretched to its limits in a voluntary effort to accomplish
something difficult and worthwhile.
MIHALY CSIKSZENTMIHALYI, *FLOW*

As a teenager I took note of one activity I would engage in regularly that stood out from the rest: playing the piano. What was different about this activity was that I was able to lose myself in it, even though this was not always the case.

I spent the beginning portion of every practice doing warm-up exercises to strengthen my fingers. When I was learning to play a new piece, I would have to concentrate on small segments of the music until muscle memory took over and I was able to play it correctly. It was not until I had the piece memorized that I could play it without much effort. My mind would enter a meditative state, making piano playing an enjoyable activity.

My friend Pamela has a similar experience when she puts together puzzles. She can spend hours and days working on a jigsaw puzzle. When I asked her what in particular she likes about it, Pamela said she appreciates that there is one given solution to the problem and that when she has completed the puzzle she feels accomplished. Over time, she increases the challenge by assembling more difficult and larger puzzles and has created works of art by gluing the pieces together and hanging them on her wall. She delights in the process of piecing together the puzzle, the gradual emergence of the image, and the satisfaction of solving the problem.

My friend Jacob is an avid rock climber. He relishes the physical and mental challenge of scaling challenging routes. The sensation of pushing his limits, of testing his strength and endurance, brings him immense satisfaction. As he ascends a cliff face, he enters a state of flow, where time seems to slow down and his focus becomes laser sharp. The combination of physical exertion and mental concentration creates a sense of exhilaration and accomplishment that is unmatched.

When do you get the most enjoyment? Could playing piano, putting together puzzles, and rock climbing top the list? Can tasks that are not normally considered "fun" or tasks that you find difficult also be enjoyable? According to Mihaly Csikszentmihalyi, enjoyment has nothing to do with our leisure activities. Instead, enjoyment is about how immersed and challenged we feel by the task on which we are working.[1]

THE GOLDILOCKS RULE

Whether you are maniacally focused on productivity or just want to get more enjoyment from your work, flow puts you into an efficient state of mind. Getting in the flow requires that you set clear goals that are suitable for your skill level.

A few years back, I decided to play cage bingo with my two children. What struck me was how uniquely distinct our experiences were during the game.

For my then nine-year-old daughter, it was a captivating adventure. She enthusiastically called out the numbers and

FIGURE 17.1 Levels of challenge.

meticulously placed chips on her bingo card, relishing every moment of the game.

My son, who was six years old at the time, found the task of matching the called numbers with those on his card to be a delightful challenge that fully engaged his young mind.

As for me, the game had an entirely different flavor. I couldn't help but feel a sense of boredom as I simply waited to hear the next number called, just so I could place a chip on my card.

This simple game of cage bingo illustrated a profound truth: The same activity or task can evoke profoundly different experiences in individuals, depending on their unique perspectives and levels of engagement. To get into flow, you need to differentiate between different levels of challenge (figure 17.1) and find the tasks that are challenging yet completable. In other words, you have to be well matched to the task. To do this, you have to consider both task difficulty and your skill level.

When task difficulty outweighs your skill level, anxiety ensues. When the opposite is true, and the task lacks challenge given your skill level, you will likely feel bored.

THE IMPORTANCE OF FEEDBACK

Once you have a job with the right level of difficulty that keeps you challenged enough so you can stay focused without anxiety or boredom, it is time to consider how you will go about completing the required tasks. Csikszentmihalyi notes the importance of setting clear goals rather than just plugging away.[2] Often, we show up at work and try to pick up where we left off, working until it is time to go home and always feeling like there is so much more to do. Instead, we need to focus ahead of time on what we are working on specifically so that we can eliminate unnecessary distractions and activities that pull us away from our goal.

A clear goal is insufficient on its own, however. The tasks need to offer immediate feedback. When I was practicing my piano pieces, I knew when my efforts amounted to the desired outcome because I could hear the finished piece. When Pamela worked on her puzzle and a piece did not fit, that was immediate feedback that she needed to find a different piece. When she completed the puzzle, it was another source of feedback that she had followed the steps correctly. When Jacob reaches the summit, he has immediate feedback that his efforts have paid off.

Having immediate feedback lets you know whether you will get your intended results or if you need to change course. It also informs you when you are finished with that particular task. What follows a completed task is feeling a sense of accomplishment.

THE OPTIMAL EXPERIENCE

Work can sometimes feel tedious. There may be demands on your time over which you have little control and which feel unenjoyable. It may seem at times that you are keeping busy but have little to show for your efforts. As Lao Tzu said, "It's better to do nothing than to be busy with nothing."[3]

How can you attain the optimal experience of flow even under these circumstances? We explored the importance of finding tasks that are a match for your skill level and tasks that challenge you enough to help you advance. We touched on the importance of setting clear goals that provide you with immediate feedback. Now it's a matter of creating parameters that allow you to immerse yourself in the task without being sidetracked, providing you with the control you need over your actions and the opportunity to go deep into the task.

Jacob finds that a challenging climbing route is more likely to induce a state of flow than an easy one. The greater the challenge, the more focused and engaged he becomes. You need time to focus your mind. When you do so, your involvement in the task can seem effortless and your engagement will likely alter your sense of time, making it feel like it passed much more quickly.

Stretching yourself, no matter what you are working on, can help you increase your skills and you will feel more fulfilled as you accomplish greater and greater challenges. And as Csikszentmihalyi reminds us, "The purpose of the flow is to keep on flowing, not looking for a peak or utopia but staying in the flow."[4]

The main difference between *flow* and *absorption* is that when you are in flow, you have short-term peak experiences. In

---

TABLE 17.1 **Getting Into a State of Flow**

- To increase absorption in your work, set clear goals that are suitable for your skill level.
- To reduce boredom, identify more challenging tasks that you can complete, given your abilities and current knowledge.
- To manage feeling overwhelmed, identify what about the situation is most challenging.
  - If it is the size of the task, break it down into manageable chunks.
  - If it is the time frame in which you have to complete it, estimate how long you will need and ask for an extension or ask to delegate aspects of the task.
  - If the work itself is beyond your scope, get mentoring or ask to exchange the task for a more fitting one given your expertise.
  - Create a plan about how you will attain feedback about the task.
  - Eliminate distractions for a set period.

---

contrast, absorption is a more pervasive and persistent state of mind that is independent of any specific task.

CONCLUSION

It is important to know that even when you do not have control over which tasks you are given, you can enjoy your experience and feel a sense of control in the task itself. Giving yourself ample time to work without distraction is a way of controlling your environment. The rest is about controlling your internal state for an optimal experience. By matching task difficulty with your skill level, creating clear goals that provide immediate feedback, and concentrating on your task, you can reach a state of effortless involvement, one that is so enjoyable that you lose track of time.

Now that you see how attainable flow experiences can be, I will teach you two ways to increase your engagement at work, through increasing job resources and personal resources.

CHAPTER 18

Maximizing Job Resources

Every job has both demands and resources, and depending on their ratio they can be in balance or bring about burnout. Job demands are aspects of the work "that drain energy, such as work overload, conflicts with others, and future job insecurity."[1] Job resources, on the other hand, include ways that help you achieve your goals, handle the demands, and increase personal growth.

To illustrate what is meant by job resources, we will examine criteria from Wilmar Schaufeli's assessment, the Energy Compass, which is based on the Job Demands–Resources Model (figure 18.1).[2]

According to the Energy Compass, there are four categories of job resources: social, work, organizational, and developmental.

SOCIAL RESOURCES

Social resources include social support, having clarity on your role and responsibilities, and getting recognized for your efforts.

Part of the reason why social support leads to higher engagement is that it sends a message that the company for which you work cares about your well-being. One basic premise in demonstrating this principle is keeping stress levels down and encouraging work-life balance. To achieve this, your company

FIGURE 18.1 Job resources according to the Energy Compass. *Source*: Schaufeli, "Applying the Job Demands–Resources Model."

may need to increase staff size and allow you more flexibility in terms of work arrangements.

When it comes to social support such as informal mentoring, findings point to insignificant results that do little to protect you from burnout.[3] However, when provided formal mentorship, so long as there is a good fit between the mentor and the mentee, the relationship can act as a buffer for stress.[4] Mentoring reduces fatigue, increases confidence, and thereby improves self-efficacy, a primary factor for engagement.

As an example of how mentoring can make a huge difference, I refer back to Julio, the worker who is trying to keep up with the heavy demands of his job by working around the clock. Perhaps one reason Julio is overly engaged or engaged-exhausted is because he feels alone in the pursuit of his work. Maybe he is focused on tasks that are outside his scope, which is why it takes him longer to complete them. If Julio were provided mentorship by his company, his mentor might help him to understand his strengths and weaknesses and how to align his tasks accordingly. He could learn to focus on his skill set, and as a result new opportunities might become available to him.

Julio's mentor may also have far-reaching connections to experts who can help Julio home in on specific skills of interest. By having a mentor or role model, Julio will feel that the work he is doing is more meaningful, which will not only be beneficial for his company but will also improve his professional development.

When Julio feels overwhelmed by stress, his mentor might help him use different and more effective coping mechanisms. By learning how to adapt to challenging situations and by feeling like he has a sounding board in his mentor, Julio will feel supported, which will lift up his mood, his energy, and his focus and help him engage with his work even in the face of stress.[5]

If you are like Julio, you need to be clear about expectations related to your role. Too often, organizations go through management changes where such details fall through the cracks. When workers get promoted or start a new project, they may also experience a lack of clarity. Taking the time to define your role and communicate about it can have a significant positive impact.

Lastly, it is best if your employer has systems in place for you to attain recognition from your boss and colleagues about your work. If your place of work lacks feedback structures, consider what would help you feel more recognized for your efforts and suggest the adoption of these supportive new practices.

WORK RESOURCES

Work resources include how much control you feel you have over your work or how well you fit with your work environment.

In the introduction to this book, I discussed the importance of control in minimizing burnout, especially when demands are high. We will examine "fit" from the perspective of personality and skill level.

One common personality trait that researchers have studied with relationship to burnout is the introversion-extroversion dimension. An introvert is someone who turns inward to recharge. Samantha is an introvert and after a long day at the office spending time in meetings, interacting with coworkers, and dealing with customers, she is ready to plop down on the couch with a glass of wine, listen to some relaxing music, and decompress from her day. Being around others is energy depleting for Samantha. She seeks ways to recharge that reverse this equation.

Part of the reason Samantha becomes drained at work is that she needs to spend time alone to think. When she is in meetings having to make decisions, she has to participate in an extroverted world. Being in a leadership position requires Samantha to be outward facing, but this is exhausting because she would prefer to be in the background rather than at the forefront. Because she is subject to overstimulation, she will more likely procrastinate to avoid additional stress.

An extrovert is someone who requires contact with others to feel an energetic charge. Whereas Samantha wants to turn down the noise, Eric, who is an extrovert, prefers to reach out to a friend to talk things over. When Eric sits alone on the train on his way to work or sits at his computer for too long, he suffers because what he needs most is human interaction.

Extroverts like Eric are outgoing and talkative. They enjoy the fast-paced job environments, the type of work that will lead introverts to more easily burn out. During meetings, extroverts do well in brainstorming sessions because they think out loud.

It is just how their brain processes information. When extroverts are in a leadership position, they relish being at center stage.

In addition to control and fit, a third work resource is your task variety. If you engage in a singular activity or in several tasks that are not varied from each other, you are likely to feel bored and become disengaged.

ORGANIZATIONAL RESOURCES

Your employer has additional resources by which to promote engagement. These include communication, trust and fairness, and values that are congruent with your own.

Communication and clarity are essential for the company goals to be understood and achieved by their employees. You need to clearly understand the expectations of you, what you need to do to achieve your goals, and how your part contributes to the overall vision of the company.

Companies create trust in their leadership by implementing strategies that tackle potential conflicts, provide a safe and nurturing environment, and bring team members together. Christine Porath, a professor at the McDonough School of Business at Georgetown University, found that when you feel respected at work, your focus and engagement increase.[6] She encourages companies to provide friendly work environments, including among coworkers. She says this can be achieved by "thanking people, sharing credit, listening attentively, humbly asking questions, acknowledging others, and smiling."[7]

Since unfair treatment is one of the factors associated with a job-person mismatch, and ultimately burnout, it follows that fairness on the job would lead to engagement. Fairness can include the work environment, flexibility of work schedules, diversity of staff, as well as decisions about pay and advancement.[8]

Another job-person mismatch is related to values. Ensure your values are similar to those of the organization so you can feel committed to your work.

DEVELOPMENTAL RESOURCES

Developmental resources include feedback, opportunities for learning and development, and career perspective.

Feedback is essential for you to be able to fine-tune your performance. While it is true that you came to the job with a particular skill set, you must fit into the company culture and need guidance about how to tweak your actions accordingly.

It is advisable for the company to provide opportunities for you to grow, not only to help you develop new skills that can enhance the company's success but to hold onto you as an employee. Without challenge, there is a risk of under-engagement.

For you to meet goals more efficiently and effectively over time, the company can invest in programs that tackle common skill-related deficiencies (e.g., time management and emotional intelligence). The benefits of this are twofold. The company will get better results and keep you there longer, while you will attain personal and professional growth on the job and be less negatively affected by stress.

You must have a roadmap for your career, and this is something the company can develop as a way of motivating you to stay working there and move up the ranks. Research conducted for the book *Good to Great* demonstrates that building leadership

TABLE 18.1   Obtaining Job Resources

Consider the questions below and what you can do to increase social resources, work-life balance, and your professional development while taking into account your organizational culture.

Social Resources

☐ *Mentorship*: Do you have a mentor to guide your professional development?

☐ *Recognition*: Do you receive recognition from colleagues and clients for your work?

☐ *Clear Expectations*: Do you understand the expectations for your role?

Work-Life Balance

☐ *Autonomy*: Do you have control over aspects of your work, such as your schedule or workload?

☐ *Job Fit*: Does your job align with your skills, interests, and values?

☐ *Task Variety*: Do you have a diverse range of tasks to keep you engaged?

☐ *Work-Life Balance*: Do you have flexibility in your schedule to balance work and personal life?

Professional Development

☐ *Performance Feedback*: Do you receive regular feedback on your performance and areas for improvement?

☐ *Career Development*: Does the company provide opportunities for professional growth and advancement?

Organizational Culture

☐ *Company Vision*: Do you understand the company's mission and goals?

☐ *Clear Expectations*: Do you know what is expected of you in your role?

☐ *Contribution*: Do you see how your role contributes to the company's success?

☐ *Conflict Resolution*: Are conflicts addressed and resolved effectively?

☐ *Positive Environment*: Does your workplace foster a positive, supportive, and inclusive culture?

☐ *Fairness*: Do you believe that decisions about pay, promotions, and opportunities are fair?

☐ *Value Alignment*: Do your personal values align with the company's values?

from within the organization is better for business than searching for outsiders to lead.[9]

Each organization needs to assess its various job resources to determine which ones to improve on to tackle engagement and burnout.

CONCLUSION

Demands are part of any job. To avoid being drained by them, you need to have access to resources. Social support, control, communication, and feedback are examples of different types of job resources that can help you get the job done. By accessing social, work, organizational, and developmental resources, you will ensure you are clear about your role, are well matched for the job, and have a roadmap for continued growth.

CHAPTER 19

Leveraging Personal Resources

While you may have little control over job resources, I will explain how personal resources are ways you can increase engagement. Mindset plays a big part in mitigating stress. Personal resources, also known as "psychological capital," are the within-person capacities, or the four pillars of hope, efficacy, resilience, and optimism (HERO).[1] These pillars correspond with increased life and job satisfaction, and by focusing on them you can augment your personal resources. Having psychological capital can help you feel confident to take on challenges, persevere, and bounce back. Developing even a single one of these pillars will likely increase the other three.

HOPE

Hope is a form of positive thinking based on realistic optimism and includes expectations that good things will happen. Researchers suggest that hope is linked to goals as well as to plans to meet those goals.[2] In other words, when you want to accomplish something you maintain your motivation through the belief that your goal is attainable and seek pathways to that goal.

What sets hope apart from mere optimism is its dynamic nature. While optimism alone may involve maintaining a positive attitude, hope takes things a step farther. Hopeful individuals are not just passive believers in a brighter future; they are action oriented. They anticipate potential obstacles and, with a strategic mindset, develop plans to navigate around them. Hope, therefore, encompasses a proactive approach to problem-solving and goal attainment.

The depth of your hope is closely tied to your level of awareness and understanding of the situations you encounter. Those who possess a comprehensive understanding of their circumstances are better equipped to gauge their own capabilities and assess the feasibility of their goals. Alternatively, some individuals may choose to remain in the dark or dismiss pertinent information, their outlook clouded by a reluctance to embrace reality. Consequently, their approach to overcoming challenges becomes fragmented.[3]

You may feel hopeful but have a distorted sense of reality, in which case you are just wishful. This sort of hope is not action-oriented and is therefore similar to plain optimism. It is false hope.

On the flip side, when your perception aligns with a grim reality, a sense of hopelessness may set in. This typically occurs when you fully grasp the difficulties you're facing and believe the situation is beyond your control. In such instances, hopelessness takes hold, leading to a passive resignation to circumstances. This state of helplessness can be particularly prominent in cases of burnout, where you might feel utterly drained and devoid of energy to take any action.

In *Good to Great*, Jim Collins shares the paradoxical story of Jim Stockdale, an American military officer who, while held captive for eight years during the Vietnam War, never lost faith that he would prevail.[4] Stockdale made it out alive, but not all of his prison mates did. What is paradoxical is that, according to Stockdale, those who felt most optimistic were the ones who did not make it out alive.

The optimists in Stockdale's group kept imagining they would get out by a specific date. When time and again that did not come to pass, they reportedly died of a broken heart.

The lesson from the Stockdale Paradox is that to be truly resilient you have to face your challenges, not wish them away. You must remain realistic and focus on aspects of the challenge over which you have control. In Stockdale's case he focused on lifting the morale of his fellow prisoners, and by focusing on something he had control over, he persevered.

Whether you are feeling more and more hopeless or have lost your hope entirely, it is essential to find a way out. Sometimes you may opt for a passive stance because you worry about disappointment, but this is dangerous territory that can lead to depression. Instead, remember that when situations are outside of your control you need to focus on acceptance and on managing your emotions.

Do you tend to catastrophize when something goes wrong? Do you tell yourself that "things will never change" or that "this always happens"? Pay attention to extreme language. Usage of words like "always" and "never" makes you believe that you have less control than you do and that difficulties are permanent. Instead, think of exceptions to the rule, times when this challenge either was not present and circumstances were better or when you were able to overcome it. This helps you remember that even when there are obstacles, they are temporary, and that when barriers are permanent, the way you think about those obstacles can still shift.

To develop real (as opposed to false) hope, you need to have something exciting to look forward to in the near or distant future. This goal is something that you believe you can accomplish due to your agency (efficacy) and pathway (resources). Throughout this discussion of developing hope, I draw on the work of Fred Luthans and colleagues, which highlights several ways to develop hope at work.[5]

Having goals is an essential criterion to develop hope because it highlights where you are currently, where you want to go, and how to get there. When you are clear on why you have your goals, your involvement takes on more meaning and increases your motivation to work.

When developing your goals, ensure they are specific rather than generic. For example, if you want to make more money, stating your intent in this way does not specify how much more you want to make and therefore does not let you know when you have reached that goal. If, instead, you specified you want to get a 10 percent raise in salary, now you have a set number in mind that you can work toward.

Goals must also be measurable. How will you know, otherwise, when you have succeeded? By being clear on ways that you can track your progress and what the end outcome will look or feel like, you increase your chances for success.

Stretch goals are goals that are challenging and allow for growth and increased engagement but are still achievable. In addition to the simple goals you might be working toward, you want to incorporate goals that stretch you beyond your limits. Referring back to the goal of making more money, a simple goal might be to make an extra thousand dollars while a stretch goal might be to double your income.

When you formulate your goals, state them in ways that are positive in terms of what you will do rather than about what you will refrain from doing. Instead of saying, "To save money, I will not go out to eat during the week," you will have more success if you say, "I will cook my meals during the week and invest the extra money that I save in my retirement account."

Sometimes goals feel overwhelming, especially those stretch goals. To maintain your hopeful framework, break your goals down into smaller milestones and focus on the little steps you can take to make progress toward your bigger goals.

When a car drives over a patch of grass in the exact same location day after day, it creates a visible path. The same happens in your brain when you do something over and over again, whether you do it outright or only in your mind. The latter technique is called *mental rehearsal*, and it has been shown to light up the same parts of the brain as actually doing the activity.

While it is true that your past experiences can be useful lessons for how to accomplish your future goals, it is best to think about new possibilities rather than just limiting your solutions to ones you have already tried. Try mentally rehearsing the steps you will take to achieve your goals. This improves your pathway thinking.

Even when you are excited about a goal you are working toward, there are times when you can lose momentum. To this end, it is helpful to build habits that sustain your motivation. For example, create a morning ritual that you do when you wake up. Start each day by visualizing your goal and meditating on the next steps you need to take in order to achieve it. By habituating a specific behavior that you want to engage in at a particular time, you create a sustainable practice for success.

When you work for someone else, creating goals is not enough. There are additional pieces to the puzzle for which you will need cooperation from your company. Because you do not operate in a vacuum, you need the support of upper management. They can empower you by giving you increased auto-

TABLE 19.1 Ways to Cultivate More Hope at Work

In your notebook, answer the following questions to set yourself up for success at work. This planning session will help you identify areas to target to increase engagement.

How can I think about my situation realistically and optimistically?

_____

_____

What are specific and measurable goals that I hope to accomplish?

_____

_____

What are my achievable stretch goals?

_____

_____

What plans do I have about how to accomplish those goals?

_____

_____

What obstacles might I encounter in pursuit of these goals?

_____

_____

Do I have a contingency plan in place for how to tackle obstacles?

_____

_____

What aspects of the work do I have control over?

_____

_____

What aspects of the work don't I have control over? How is this affecting me? (Remember to focus on acceptance and emotional management.)

_____

_____

Instead of catastrophizing or giving up, what are exceptions to the rule or more helpful ways of thinking about the situation? (Remember that obstacles are usually temporary.)

_____

_____

Am I focusing on what I will do rather than what I will avoid?

_____

_____

What are the identifiable milestones for my goals?

_____

_____

Have I mentally rehearsed the steps I will take?

_____

_____

Do I have habits in place to sustain my motivation?

_____

_____

Do I want to ask for more autonomy to make decisions, delegate, and participate in new opportunities?

_____

_____

Am I getting recognized for my actions?

_____

_____

Am I getting positive feedback about my work?

_____

_____

Do I understand what is expected of me?

_____

_____

Are my strengths and talents aligned with available resources?

_____

_____

nomy to make decisions and delegate so you have more time to participate in new opportunities. They can provide recognition as well as positive feedback, which explains how your actions are directly tied to the outcome of the company. Employees often do not get to see the direct results of their hard work, so having this feedback can be very motivating to continue on your course. When you are setting goals, your manager can help align your strengths and talents with appropriate resources. Lastly, the leadership team can provide you with hands-on training focused on developing your talents into strengths.

No matter where you are currently on the burnout spectrum, you can develop hope through these methods. Aim to have a realistic grasp of the situation in front of you and maintain a hopeful outlook that leads you to anticipate obstacles, create plans around them, and attain your goals. Make sure your goals are clear, challenging, and attainable and that you enlist the support and resources needed for success. This can quickly improve your outlook and experience.

Believing that change is possible directly ties into your belief in your ability to make the change. The latter is your self-efficacy belief.

EFFICACY

If you really do put a small value upon yourself, rest assured that the world will not raise your price.
ANONYMOUS

From Perceived Failure to Extraordinary Success

At the age of 28, Joanne saw herself as a failure. After her marriage fell apart, she was an unemployed single mom and so poor that she had to receive welfare benefits. She fell into a deep depression.

Joanne could have stayed stuck in a negative state of mind, thinking about life's disappointments, comparing herself to more successful friends, or telling herself that she would never climb out of the pit in which she found herself.

But Joanne was determined to be a writer. She would spend her days pushing her baby's stroller, and once her infant daughter fell asleep Joanne would sit in a cafe and write. It took her two years, but she ultimately finished her first book.

With her manuscript in hand, Joanne then faced rejection after rejection. In total, 12 publishing houses turned her down. Two years after the book's completion, one publisher finally agreed to print a limited run of only 1,000 copies of the book. That decision changed the course of history.

Within five months of publishing, Joanne's book earned several awards and was picked up by a major multinational publisher who paid her $105,000. Joanne now had recognition as a writer and the financial security to continue her craft.

Joanne's success started with an idea and was attained through determination, patience, and a strong belief in her abilities despite the odds. She is widely known as J. K. Rowling, the author of the Harry Potter book series, whose brand is now worth an estimated $15 billion.

The Power of Belief

It is one thing to believe that change is possible and another to make it happen. If you want to change your financial situation you might buy a lottery ticket and hope to win a lot of money. There is a minuscule chance that you will find success with this strategy. Alternatively, you can ask yourself, "What can I do to create financial increases in my life?" This is a more powerful approach over which you have control.

The belief in your ability to succeed, which drives you to face challenges even when you may have failed in the past, is called self-efficacy. Your efficacy belief determines the amount of effort you invest. The more you invest of yourself, the higher the chances that you will be successful.

Multiple factors affect your belief in your abilities. If, for instance, you are asked to give a presentation at work in front of your entire division, your response may vary greatly depending on your *history*. If you have never spoken in front of a group or have tried it before but feel you had failed miserably, you will see yourself as less competent, which will negatively affect your efficacy in this task. Alternatively, if you have previously mastered public speaking, you will likely believe that you will succeed in this task, thereby increasing your efficacy. Thus, it is not the task itself that determines your belief but rather your associations with that task based on personal experiences that influence how you perceive it.

Even if you're new to your position and have no prior experience, you can increase your efficacy by watching other people perform the task at hand, what is referred to as *vicarious learning*. Research has shown that when we observe those who are similar to us engaging in a particular behavior, we overcome our fears more rapidly and believe that we too can be successful.[6]

A less powerful influence that can alter your efficacy is *verbal persuasion*. If you are feeling doubtful about your ability to succeed in a task, sometimes all it takes is encouragement from your boss, coworker, or friend to give you the boost you need to get started. The reason this method is not as reliable is that it can also work against you. If you are not highly efficacious and someone discourages you by pointing out the likelihood of failure or the difficulty ahead, your belief in your ability to succeed will likely diminish further.

Had J. K. Rowling not believed as staunchly as she did in her writing, she might have felt hopeless about being able to change her depressing life. Had she internalized the dozen rejections she received when trying to publish her manuscript, she might have given up entirely. Even though Rowling had never published a book before, she did not let this challenge frighten her. She was able to sustain her energy no matter what the outside world presented because of her strong self-efficacy. Like Rowling, if you believe enough in yourself, you will be able to attain your goals with determination. By pushing yourself to achieve tasks that are unfamiliar and challenging, you can reach even greater heights.

In addition to history, vicarious learning, and verbal persuasion, there is another factor that can influence your belief in your ability. When you are faced with challenges, your body might experience physical arousal. If you interpret that arousal as unfavorable, you will be filled with fear and either avoid the project or sabotage your efforts. Alternatively, when you reframe your arousal as excitement, you can use the momentum of your inner state to delve into the task.

As you can see, low efficacy beliefs are associated with threats to be avoided while high efficacy beliefs are linked to challenges to be mastered. Because of these associations it is easy to see how your beliefs can lead to self-fulfilling prophecies. Self-discouragement leads to avoidance, which prevents you from experiencing success and reinforces the belief that you are unable to successfully tackle a particular task. Conversely, self-encouragement leads to an investment of effort and higher chances of success, which furthers your belief in your ability.

Your self-talk can either lead you to spiral out of control or into a state of flow.

How Beliefs Affect Performance

Sometimes in life you will be faced with extreme challenges. These challenges may be external (e.g., high demands or a shortage of resources) or internal, including a negative state of mind. Regardless of the source of your main challenges, remain aware of how they affect you and take control of your reactions.

If you have ever had a "bad day," you might recall how a single negative event set the tone, making you anticipate further unfavorable outcomes. The more you focused on negative outcomes, the more you found yourself attracting adverse events to you.

On the flip side, you may have had the experience of a "winning streak" in which you experienced something favorable that put you in a very optimistic mood. For the rest of that day, you anticipated winning and consequently found a parking spot right in front of the grocery store, found money on the street, or got promoted at your job.

Sometimes these streaks last more than a day. We see this in people who experience clinical depression. They can stay stuck in a negative thought pattern for weeks, months, or even years. They become so convinced they cannot win that their mood becomes part of their identity.

Even throughout your day, you might have ups and downs, not only in your mood or way of thinking but in your perception of your ability to be successful. Reflect on this scenario: Equipped with your existing skills, you enter your place of work, where you have specific resources. Given your view of yourself based on past experiences and that of your environment, you form an initial judgment of your ability to complete the task at hand.

You notice anxiety forming. This happens whenever you feel less confident about what is asked of you, usually when the task is unfamiliar, complex, or one where you have failed in the past and have not yet learned from that failure. Whenever you experience anxiety, you cannot help but feel wary about taking action. Despite this hesitation, you plunge ahead but are ultimately unsuccessful.

Should this scenario happen without you either figuring out what you did wrong so you can self-correct or without specific, accurate, and timely feedback from your manager, you will be left guessing. Given the little information you have, you may come up with an incorrect explanation for your failure.

With each repetition of this scenario, your confidence decreases, which directly affects your performance. If you continue experiencing failure after failure, you might conclude that your lack of success is due to your inadequacies, bad luck, or to not having enough control over the situation. You might start labeling yourself as a "loser" and become increasingly anxious or frustrated. This will further decrease your belief in your ability to succeed.

A streak of poor performances despite your efforts can lead you to process information automatically about failures and lack of successes and, perhaps, to expect future failure. This can cause such strong anxiety that you might procrastinate to avoid the pain of another anticipated disappointment.

TABLE 19.2   **Increasing Efficacy**

To create patience, determination, and a strong belief in your abilities despite any odds:

- watch others perform the task to learn from them.
- talk to your manager for affirmation that you can successfully tackle this task.
- interpret physical signs of arousal as excitement rather than fear.
- ask for specific, accurate, and timely feedback.
- when you aren't successful, objectively assess why not.
- avoid labeling yourself a loser.
- maintain a positive mindset even in the face of failures.
- stay in action mode. Confidence is not built from passivity.

This scenario demonstrates a downward spiral. Beliefs play a significant role in your performance, and without adequate information in the form of feedback it is tempting to fall into the trap of wrongly attributing your failures to your inadequacies. This only further complicates the situation, and you perpetuate a sense of despair. Knowing this, you can be mindful of your self-talk and seek out objective data that can help you analyze the challenge, giving you a different perspective and pointing to new directions to tackle. In chapter 21 you will learn more about how to break down your experience so you can gain insight into what starts and maintains a spiral, as well as how to stop and reverse it. These insights can increase your chances of success and decrease your failure rate.

RESILIENCE

Our greatest glory is not in never falling,
but in rising every time we fall.
CONFUCIUS

Part of what makes jumping on trampolines so much fun is that when you apply pressure, the springs help you shoot up. Resilience is like a spring: it is your ability to bounce back from adversity.

We are all resilient to a point. Think about all the disappointments, failures, and defeats you have encountered in your life. If you were not resilient, you would not be able to keep going. So when you come across a disappointment or a harsh reality, how do you get past it? What is the process you go through that allows you to bounce back? As it turns out, the keys are in your biology and your mind.

The Biology of Resilience

Charles Darwin highlighted a theory to explain why some people thrive while others wither away, which he named the "Survival of the Fittest." In this evolutionary theory, Darwin described the process of natural selection. When the going gets tough, the tough get going, leaving the not-so-tough in a cloud of smoke. He attributed the differences between these two different types of people to their genes.[7]

Research and history have demonstrated that there is truth to this theory. People with family histories of mental illness are more likely to experience mental illness themselves. People with family histories of medical illnesses, such as type 1 diabetes, cancer, or heart disease, are more likely to experience such diseases in their lifetime.

That being said, with the advancement of science and medicine, we have been able to give never-before-seen advantages to the biologically predisposed. Even if your father and his father suffered from lifelong depression, when you struggle with depression there are more medications and treatments today than ever that can help you overcome this illness. The more we know about the brain and the mind, the more we realize that there is also a lot you can do to help yourself.

The Psychology of Resilience

Psychologist Carole Dweck made popular the notion of a growth versus a fixed mindset.[8] According to her, when faced with an obstacle, people with a growth mindset can counterbalance negative events by focusing on their positive aspects. If your company suddenly announces major layoffs and you lose your job, if you hold a growth mindset you will likely stay optimistic and focus on finding a new one. If, however, you have a fixed mindset, you might attribute the loss to a personal attribute and consequently feel depressed and unmotivated to pursue another position.

There are multiple layers to your mind. Like an onion, the core of your mind lies in the center and is hardest to change. This core determines the direction of the layers that come after it. That innermost layer is comprised of your *schema* or *core beliefs.*

The lens through which you each see the world makes up the core beliefs you hold to be true, even in the face of evidence to the contrary. These beliefs lead you to attribute causality to internal, stable, and global factors, which can turn out to be what are known as *attribution errors.*

Like the child who blames herself for her parent's actions, we as adults might attribute events to three factors that make us less resilient. The first is an *internal factor*. If you have a fixed mindset, you are likely to attribute the layoff to something deficient in yourself. This often stems from a core belief that you are inadequate. When you believe this, you tend to look for evidence that demonstrates you are right. Therefore, when something happens, such as losing your job, you are more likely to blame yourself.

The second factor that reduces our resilience is the *stability* factor. When you believe that your flaw is permanent, you are less likely to feel optimistic about your ability to bounce back. Not only do you see yourself as inadequate, but you feel hopeless about being able to change that inadequacy.

Finally, the third factor that makes people less resilient in the face of stress is a global one. When you have shortcomings, you can see them as weaknesses. If, instead, you think of yourself as the problem, you are taking a local problem (the shortcoming) and making a global issue out of it. When you do this, every failure reinforces your belief that you are a failure. This belief is not only accompanied by feelings of shame but also makes you less likely to keep trying. This is sometimes why people become stuck.

Do you believe you are not enough? This limiting core belief is part of a fixed mindset that can lead you to misattribute your inadequacies to everything that goes wrong, especially if you believe you cannot overcome your limitations. Instead of feeling guilty when you make a mistake, you feel ashamed of yourself. In this case, work on rewiring your brain to change your limiting belief. Affirm that you are enough often and with consistency until you build the habit and neural pathways in your brain to believe it is true. Doing so will help you put events into perspective and recognize that when something falls short of expectation, it is a specific rather than a global aspect that went awry. Remember the adage, "Don't throw the baby out with the bathwater."

In Search of Meaning

If you were one of Jim Stockdale's prison mates in the Vietnam War, what would allow you to accept your harsh reality when what you want most is to be free? As previously mentioned, the way you think about your situation can mean the difference between life and death.

Viktor Frankl was also a prisoner; he was imprisoned in a Nazi concentration camp during World War II. Frankl survived and subsequently wrote *Man's Search for Meaning*. In the book he explains what allowed him to survive. For Frankl it was about finding a purpose and imagining his desired outcome; by doing so, he could feel positive, even in the midst of his dire circumstances.[9]

According to Frankl, all prisoners experienced shock, which over time led to apathy and eventually to depersonalization.

This is not all that different from the cycle of burnout. The stress experienced from the high demands of your job leads you to overexert yourself. Over time you become worn out and cynical.

What is so radical about Frankl's philosophy is that he contends that there is meaning in everything, even in suffering and death. This is in line with the HERO dimensions of psychological capital. Without meaning you lose all resilience of mind.

Maladaptive Coping

Coping is the way we respond when faced with a situation. There are three maladaptive ways of coping. I will teach you how to classify your behaviors based on these coping styles so you can focus on adaptive and more balanced ways of coping instead.

Imagine that you believe you are not lovable. If your preferred coping style is one of *overcompensation*, you might find yourself becoming a people pleaser. Deep down, you think that people will love you only if you make them happy, so you dance circles around others' needs while ignoring your own. From an energetic perspective, when you overly exert yourself, you are overutilizing your energy.

The second type of maladaptive coping is *avoidance*. Rather than doing or feeling too much, you run away from the problem. If you find yourself saying, "I just don't want to think about it," you are avoiding your reality. The issue with this model is that the problem will not just go away. You might be able to distract your mind for the moment and opt for immediate gratification, but sooner or later the problem resurfaces. Often when you face a problem that you believe is out of your control and one that may be too painful to focus on, you try to cover it up. This can lead to developing bad habits (e.g., addictions).

The third type of poor coping you want to be aware of is *surrendering*. This coping happens when you believe your flaws are global. You think there is nothing you can do, so you give up trying; you accept that you are doomed for failure. From an energy perspective this represents an internal collapse or deficiency. Returning to my previous example, if you believe you are not lovable, rather than try to win people over, you might isolate yourself and fall into a depression.

Adaptive Coping: Tipping the Scale of Resiliency

To some degree, your genes and learned behaviors affect the way you respond to stress, but this does not mean there is nothing you can do to help yourself. You can focus on learning skills that help you face challenges and override your ineffective automatic responses so that you can be more in control. You can appraise situations more accurately rather than blame yourself when you are not exclusively responsible. When you become highly emotional, you can ground yourself and think through the situation once more when your mind is clear. Rather than revert to sugar, drugs, alcohol, or any other substance to change your state, focus on healthy alternatives. Ultimately, the goal is to face your challenges, not run away from them, but when emotions run high, find effective ways of managing them first, then come back to problem-solving.

Instead of looking at your deficiencies, improve on your weaknesses or accept them and look to your strengths. Effort counts. Focus on what you want more of, not on what you don't want.

Social Support

Your relationships also help your resilience. Who are your cheerleaders? When you are struggling, is there anyone who will give you encouragement to keep going even when it seems all the odds are stacked against you? Build your support team. This can consist of friends, family members, teachers, therapists, or coaches. You may also feel inspired by fictional characters in a movie you saw or a book you read. Your support person may be a celebrity or someone you admire. Once you have located your squad, know that you can rely on their support in tough times, even if only in your mind. If your support team consists of deceased individuals or people you cannot contact, internalize their voice, and when faced with a challenge, ask yourself what they would say. Remember, being vulnerable is not a sign of weakness. It is much more beneficial to have the courage to know your limitations and ask for support when you need it.

If you do not feel you have a support team, even having just one person on your side can make you more resilient. If you need to increase your circle, look for like-minded individuals. Consider volunteer opportunities or a place of worship to create community. Call people who do not live close to you. Technology is helping us break distance and financial barriers to communication. And if being around others is too overwhelming, you can gain similar benefits from having a pet.

Knowing what affects you most and preparing for it in advance can help you stay grounded in the presence of stress. Reflect on past mistakes and the lessons you have gleaned. Try to visualize what happened, and rather than seeing yourself respond the same way, replace your response by applying these lessons learned. Notice how different the outcome will be with these new applications. By visualizing a positive outcome you are prepping yourself for a more favorable one the next time around.

According to John Boyd and Philip Zimbardo, authors of *The Time Paradox*, individuals who are positive about past events tend to be more resilient. When they bring to mind memories from the past, they think of those events in an optimistic way.

The authors note a correlation between the way these individuals think about their past and their current mental state. They tend to experience less anger, anxiety, and depression.[10]

While resilience is about maintaining your integrity during a big change, adaptability allows you to adjust to the situation or at least have a different perspective.

Adaptability

When I was growing up, my family did not have the same financial means as many of my friends. While kids in my class focused on certain brands of clothes or shoes that were fashionable, as an eight-year-old I had to contend with more significant issues. I was a recent immigrant who arrived in the United States without knowledge of the English language. I was put in a classroom with American students and primarily expected to fit in, but I did not.

For the majority of my first year I could not even understand what people around me were saying. Eventually I was able to formulate sentences in English, but I still felt so inadequate and shy that I tried to blend in rather than stand out. I desperately wanted to feel normal. Even if mimicking behaviors of others made no sense, it was my attempt at being like everyone else.

So in the years following my arrival to the States, when my classmates were fashion conscious and keeping up with the Joneses became their favorite pastime, I had to rationalize to myself that having knockoffs was a good alternative. I convinced myself that being different is part of what makes me unique.

I will be the first to admit that being an outsider was not easy at the time. It led to feelings of loneliness and inadequacy, but it also provided me with something else that contributed to my character.

Because at a young age I had to jump through hoops, face difficult challenges, and think about who I was in comparison to those around me, I became resilient. I could not take many things for granted. I had to redefine normal. I had to make up my own rules. I had to rediscover myself.

After attending the same elementary school for five years, I attended a summer camp with an entirely different group of kids. This experience served as a profound wake-up call. The children at the camp welcomed me with genuine curiosity, and to my surprise I felt a sense of being truly liked for the first time in my life. It was during that transformative summer that I had a revelation: There was absolutely nothing wrong with me, and I could wholeheartedly embrace my uniqueness. I recognized that this newfound, positive perspective was not an intrinsic change within me but rather a reflection of the empowering influence of my changed environment.

I notice my resilience in my attitude toward challenges now as an adult. My childhood experiences, which forced me to think for myself and learn to survive by adapting to my environment, helped build up my resilience muscle. My attitude of hope when faced with failure or disappointment and belief in my abilities even when faced with new tasks, coupled with an optimistic framework, allow me to persevere and ultimately reach great heights.

Building Up Your Resilience

Nan Henderson and Mike Milstein describe two ways in which you can build resilience into the work environment.[11] The first involves creating a resilient environment characterized by opportunities for meaningful engagement, clear and achievable expectations, and a culture of care and support. The second method focuses on reducing risk factors by promoting social connections, establishing well-defined boundaries, and imparting essential life skills.

Given that you likely do not have control over your work environment when you are job searching, try to find a position that promotes collaboration, provides you opportunities to progress, and supports you through feedback, rewards, or other forms of recognition. While in your position, create bonds with your coworkers, learn to work within the boundaries of the organization while setting your own boundaries, and develop your interpersonal skills to reduce conflict and increase cooperation.

Resilient people believe that things happen for a reason. They find meaning in everything rather than fixating on a specific ideal. They view setbacks as temporary and reframe them to mean an opportunity for growth. They think of themselves as stronger with each adversity they overcome rather than as helpless victims.

Resilience is a self-perpetuating cycle. The more resilient you are, the stronger you become after a negative experience. Your resilience becomes evident when you face challenging situations, not only in the way that you interpret and react to the challenges but also in your ability to adapt to change.[12]

As in the tale of the Tortoise and the Hare, resilience is not about speed;[13] it is about having the mindset and skill set to continue the journey. Arrogance is what led the hare to get off course and lose the race to a tortoise who persisted even with the knowledge of how unlikely it would be to finish ahead of a much faster animal.

When you boil it all down, the heart of the matter is trust in yourself. You have to be able to trust yourself to problem-solve and to know that even though you are imperfect, you can improve over time with the right intention and mindset.

TABLE 19.3 Strengthening Your Resilience Muscle

- View setbacks as temporary and reframe them as opportunities for growth.
- Think of yourself as growing stronger with each adversity you face.
- Cultivate a positive outlook.
- Face your challenges.
- Override automatic negative thinking.
- Improve areas of weakness or accept them and focus instead on your strengths.
- Internalize the voice of your social support team and ask yourself what they would do in your place.
- Enlarge your social circle.
- Connect regularly with supportive people who live at a distance.
- Know what affects you most and prepare in advance for your reaction.
- Review past mistakes and visualize yourself implementing new lessons.
- Focus on adapting to new situations.
- Set clear and consistent boundaries.

By focusing on what you can control, you can regulate your emotions and behaviors and make good choices to navigate the terrain.

As Brené Brown suggests, cultivating a resilient spirit is about letting go of "numbing and powerlessness."[14] This aligns with the concept of shifting from avoidance and surrender to adaptive coping strategies. It's essential to recognize that you possess more strength than you may realize, and that with dedication and perseverance you can enhance your resilience. Embracing vulnerability will lead you to a supportive circle of individuals who stand by your side. By accepting yourself as a flawed yet valuable human being, you'll come to understand that no matter how challenging external circumstances may become, your inner self harbors strength and inherent goodness.

OPTIMISM

If you have ever done the trust fall exercise, in which you are blindfolded and allow yourself to fall with the hope that you are caught in time, you know that it can feel scary. In essence, you have to learn to fall, take risks that may not pan out, and remain optimistic that you will be able to handle whatever comes your way. Optimism protects you from burnout. But as I mentioned, you still need to know how to face reality.

Optimism is not about being an idealist. Optimism is about taking a long hard look at the reality and not making more of it than is there. It is about trusting your ability to adapt while focusing your mind on the more positive aspects of a difficult situation.

There are many benefits to being optimistic. For one, optimists vary their coping methods.[15] You can view circumstances from various angles, and the perspective on which you focus will largely determine how you are affected. Optimists tend to focus on the more positive aspects and avoid dwelling on problems.[16] Being optimistic allows you to find meaning in negative events, stretch yourself, and therefore adjust better to adversity.[17] This does not mean that you are oblivious or in denial. Researchers have found that optimists are more knowledgeable about their health conditions and mindful of how to live a healthy lifestyle.[18] Pessimists tend to experience more depression, anxiety, and stress than their counterparts.[19] It seems that the optimist's fluidity of thought and adaptability in behavior lead to greater satisfaction, self-esteem, and psychological well-being.[20] The good news is that optimism, like many of the skills mentioned in this book, can be developed.

Focusing the Mind

I remember that after buying my first car, a Honda, I suddenly saw Hondas everywhere. Similarly, when I became a parent, I began to spot people with strollers wherever I went. And when strolling hand in hand with my husband, I started to observe numerous other couples together. These occurrences are not mere coincidences.

The reason we see evidence that confirms our experience is because we are focused on it, whereas beforehand we were not. This is called *confirmation bias*. We cannot possibly take in all the information around us. Doing so would overwhelm us. The brain is designed to help us survive, so it limits the input it takes in. What if there was a way to program your mind so that it could pick up on the information you deem necessary rather than the status quo? Well, there is.

Mindfulness is a practice that helps you develop the skill to focus the mind. Like any new skill, it needs to be learned and practiced over time. One way to build this muscle is to practice mindfulness meditation. You close your eyes, and rather than let your mind wander you set an intention to focus on one thought. You can focus on a word or phrase, on your breath, or on being neutral. The latter entails noticing whenever your mind drifts in any direction and then bringing it back to neutral. Each time you notice and return to center you are practicing mindfulness. The more you practice refocusing your mind when circumstances are calm, the more this skill will serve you when chaos ensues.

Your brain is a magnet for negativity. When you are negative, you have no trouble noticing when something goes wrong: You get stuck in traffic, you spill your coffee, you cannot fall asleep even though you are exhausted and know you have a big presentation the next morning. In this state, we tend to overlook when positive things happen. Pay attention when you wake up if the sun is shining, when your burger comes out just the way you like it, or when a stranger smiles at you as you pass them on the street. Even when we get feedback, we seem to focus on the one area for improvement rather than on the nine things we did right.

Mindfulness helps focus the mind on the present. Through this process, you can let go of the past and your expectations for what might be. Mindfulness looks reality right in the face and rolls with the punches rather than overthinking the situation. You can choose to focus on the things that go well around you so that you too can reap the benefits of optimism.

Gratitude

Being grateful is about feeling thankful for a benefit you have derived from someone or something. It is another example of how you can train your mind to focus on the positive aspect of a situation. Even on your toughest days, you can choose to find something to feel grateful about and focus on that. You can be thankful when the sun shines because of its light and warmth. You can feel gratitude for the rain because it hydrates the plants and allows them to grow. You can find value in any situation.

When you are trying to develop an optimistic mindset, gratitude can serve as your gateway. It too has associated benefits including more positive emotions, greater personal well-being, and improved relationships.[21]

Gratitude as a subject of scientific research has been studied only since the year 2000. In the short amount of time since then, the evidence has strongly shown that adopting an attitude of gratitude and engaging in exercises that strengthen this sense of appreciation provide ample mental, physical, and social benefits.

Mental Benefits

In 2016, researchers conducted a study to examine the benefits of gratitude journaling on university students seeking mental health counseling.[22] They divided participants into three groups, each of which received psychotherapy services. What differentiated these groups is the following: The first group had to write one gratitude letter weekly for three weeks to someone they know; the second group had to write about their thoughts and feelings related to negative past experiences; the third group did not receive instructions to write at all.

Researchers discovered that the group that wrote the gratitude letters showed significant improvements in mental health issues related to depression and anxiety, showing positive signs even 4 and 12 weeks after the experiment had ended.

What contributed to this significance of gratitude writing was the main finding that people who engaged in journaling about gratitude used fewer negative emotion-based words. The shift in focus from toxic emotions such as resentment, frustration, and regret occurred because these participants had focused on how other people contributed to their flourishing. This shift took them away from what otherwise might have been ruminative thinking.

Gratitude not only improves your mindset but can also boost your self-esteem. This result was found in athletes who practiced gratitude. Researchers believe that focusing on gratitude steers our mind away from social comparisons where we feel inferior to others who are more accomplished and allows us to appreciate them instead.[23]

Physical Benefits

A study conducted in 2012 found that more grateful participants experienced fewer physical aches and pains.[24] These individuals were more likely to engage in healthy activities such as a routine exercise regimen and regular medical check-ups. We might conclude that those who practice gratitude feel more positively about themselves and thus take better care of their bodies. Their self-care practices, therefore, result in better health.

Another study looked at the relationship between gratitude and sleep. The findings pointed to higher sleep quality and duration for grateful individuals. Due to the more positive mindset of practicing gratitude, they tended to engage in more positive thoughts before bed, which helped them attain improved sleep.[25]

Social Benefits

The authors of one of the measures of gratitude used in scientific studies, the Gratitude Resentment and Appreciation Test (GRAT), conceptualized gratitude with the following:

1. *Abundance mentality*: Rather than feel deprived when someone else has attained their goal, grateful individuals would see others' success as a joyous occasion and not harbor feelings of envy.

2. *Acknowledge others*: When they encounter success, grateful individuals take the time to acknowledge others' contributions to their accomplishments.

3. *Appreciate small details*: While it is easy for us to feel a surge of happiness when we accomplish great feats, grateful people can appreciate the simple aspects of day-to-day life.[26]

We can hypothesize that if you can rejoice in your success, acknowledge others for their contributions, and appreciate the small things in life, you will benefit from stronger social bonds. This is exactly what the research supports.

Researchers at the University of Kentucky found that gratitude correlated with decreased aggression toward others.[27] That is, individuals who scored higher on gratitude scales were found to have more empathy toward others and were less likely to seek revenge when something went wrong. This finding demonstrates both a social and emotional benefit in that grateful individuals are more likely to reduce interpersonal conflict and experience more social closeness with others because they are harboring less anger.

When we express our gratitude to others it deepens our interpersonal connections.[28] And as the saying goes, "You reap what you sow." When you build close relationships, you have greater access to social support when you need it. Because having these relationships decreases your stress and improves your mood, you are also less likely to need support.

Ways to Be Grateful

Now that you are aware of the prosperity associated with a gratitude practice, I will explain how you too can reap these benefits.

According to researcher Sara Algoe of the University of North Carolina, gratitude is a three-step process that she terms "Find-Remind-Bind":

- Step 1 is to *find* people with whom you are compatible.
- Step 2 is to *remind* yourself of existing social relationships.
- Step 3 is to invest in these relationships so that you can *bind* with these influential individuals.

The Find-Remind-Bind process demonstrates that gratitude is a practice that brings you into connection with other people and is an ongoing exercise that nourishes these interpersonal bonds.[29]

Consider your social circle. Are the people in it compatible with your personality and values? If you are content with the bonds you have, focus on engaging with these individuals on a deeper level. If, however, you want to increase your circle, if you want to find new and more fitting friendships, and if you want to feel less lonely and more connected with others, focus on finding the bonds first. Expand your community by joining local chapters of like-minded individuals. Consider neighborhood groups, religious organizations such as churches and temples, meditation circles, or volunteer opportunities. You can join both leisure and business networking events in your area through sites such as Meetup and Eventbrite. Create a goal and take the necessary steps to see it to fruition.

You can also focus on your inner world to reap the benefits, a practice over which you have more control and can engage in more frequently. Here are three ways to practice gratitude:

1. Write a thank-you note to someone you appreciate. Simply the act of writing such a letter invokes positive emotions in you, whether or not you send it. That said, should you have the opportunity to share your letter with the person to whom you are

grateful, this would be an exercise that can allow you to deepen your connection with that individual.

2. Start a gratitude journal. Everyday write in a notebook about what you are thankful for by focusing your mind on the positive. This will sharpen your attention to the small details of life, as mentioned above. This practice can be as short as a couple of minutes of writing, so do not let a lack of time be an excuse. Simply get in the habit of writing down three events from that day that you are grateful for and, as a bonus, consider writing your contribution to these events. If you are thankful for someone in your life, reflect on a recent occurrence that sparked this sense of appreciation in you.

3. Practice a loving-kindness meditation (Metta) daily. This type of meditation involves mentally sending goodwill, kindness, and warmth toward others by silently repeating a series of mantras, and it fosters compassion for yourself and others. It replaces self-criticism with more positivity and helps you feel more socially connected. Furthermore, it can reduce pain associated with migraines and slow down aging.[30]

Research has shown that people who take the time to reflect on and write about the good things in their life were not only more optimistic but also felt happier and more satisfied.[31] To download your free gratitude template and to access a guided loving-kindness meditation, go to www.BurnoutToResilience .com.

TABLE 19.4 **Cultivating Optimism**

Trust your ability to adapt and focus on the positive aspects of a difficult situation by following the guidelines below.

- Be open to new perspectives and possibilities.
- Use fewer negative, emotion-based words.
- Practice self-care.
- Adopt an abundance mentality.
- Celebrate other people's wins.
- Acknowledge others' contribution to your success.
- Appreciate small details.
- Find people with whom you are compatible.
- Remind yourself of existing social relationships in your life.
- Maintain and invest in those relationships.
- Every day, write down three things for which you are grateful and how you contributed to them.
- Practice loving kindness to maintain a positive mindset about others, even when they act out.

No matter where you currently find yourself, you can always cultivate a more optimistic mindset. Practice mindfulness and gratitude daily, have trust in yourself and in what is possible, and pay closer attention to the positives that show up every day in your life. What you focus on will expand.

CONCLUSION

The four pillars of psychological capital are your personal resources that can help you manage the demands of your work.

These pillars are hope, efficacy, resilience, and optimism. To-gether, they encourage you to employ positive yet realistic thinking that is action-oriented, a belief in your ability to suc-ceed, adaptability, and a sense of purpose regardless of the chal-lenges you face or the number of failures you have endured.

By embracing these pillars, you can set yourself up for suc-cess. As a result of more exceptional achievement, you will in-crease your efficacy. The more you believe in yourself, the more you will embrace challenges and adaptively cope with them. The more trials you endure, the more resilient you will become. Your growth mindset will lead to continued opportunities and greater satisfaction. Furthermore, you will establish stronger social con-nections, improve your well-being, and appreciate life more.

CHAPTER 20

Mastering Time Management

To be efficient so you can be effective, you have to consider how well you manage your time. One of the reasons people become so stressed out at work is that they feel there is more to do than there is time. This is not, by any stretch, a new dilemma. It's about how one deals with it that can make all the difference.

I have divided time management up into three segments: prioritization, procrastination, and perfect attention.

PRIORITIZATION

All too often we are swamped by the number of demands placed on us. We might even take on other people's work because they ask. Realistically, we don't have an infinite amount of time or energy, so the amount of work we take on has to match our existing resources.

While the requirements of your job may not be entirely in your hands, you have to ask yourself, "What is something that only I can do?" They hired you for a reason. You have unique talents, experiences, and abilities that differentiate you from your coworkers. What makes you unique at work? Hone in on those areas to provide maximum value.

What happens to the rest of the requests, responsibilities, and demands placed on you? This is where prioritization comes in.

If you've ever used an organization system, you know that it's essential to divide items into piles. For instance, if you were organizing shoes, you might separate athletic shoes from dress shoes or closed-toed shoes from sandals. By placing items in categories, it is easier to identify them when you need them the most.

When it comes to your work, you need to segment as well. Imagine that you have a four-part filter through which all requests get funneled (figure 20.1). As a task comes in, rather than have it pile up in a single stack, ask yourself, "Which part of the filters does it belong in?"

The first filter is for urgent and important tasks. These are tasks that you need to get done immediately. Your attention should go to these so you can clear them out. The goal here would be that once those tasks are out of the way, you keep this filter empty as much as possible. One of the reasons we burn out is because we are in a state of constant crisis. We focus on putting out fire after fire, which readily depletes our internal fire.

FIGURE 20.1 The Time Management Matrix. *Source*: Stephen R. Covey, A. Roger Merrill, and Rebecca R. Merrill, *First Things First: To Live, to Love, to Learn, to Leave a Legacy* (New York: Simon and Schuster, 1994).

Tasks that you deem essential, that only you can do, and that allow you to contribute the greatest value should go in the second filter. This is where, ideally, you spend the majority, if not all, of your time. By eliminating urgent tasks and focusing on non-urgent yet important tasks, you find higher purpose in your work without overexerting your energy. This is what allows you to enter a state of flow and feel engaged in the work.

The remaining two filters are ones to avoid as much as possible. They include tasks that are urgent but unimportant. These are tasks that someone with a lower skill set can do, such as an administrative staff person or a team member whom you are managing. They also include tasks that are non-urgent and unimportant. The reason you don't want to spend your time on these types of functions is that spending time on anything unimportant takes time away from more critical tasks.

Remember, the name of the game to being in your power, to feeling fulfilled, and to avoiding burnout is to make conscious decisions about what you are doing with your time.

Steven Covey, the author of the bestselling book *The 7 Habits of Highly Effective People*, came up with this four-quadrant system for prioritization.[1] In his experience, people who focus on urgent matters become burned out, which leads them to spend time on tasks that are neither urgent nor important. As an alternative, he suggests, plan how you will spend your time on those tasks that are important and non-urgent.

PROCRASTINATION

Sometimes, even when we need to work on a critical task, we may purposely put it off and engage in more mindless pursuits that are easier and less demanding. Why do we do this?

There are generally two answers to this question. The first is that we are burned out. When we feel energy depleted, we try to conserve energy by engaging in tasks that require less of us. When we come home tired after a day at the office, we may opt for an evening in front of the television rather than going to work out. The same can happen in the office, and we see this with superficial office banter, time spent on social media, or mindless eating.

The second reason we procrastinate is that we are unable to cope with difficult emotions, especially a fear of failure. If you are a perfectionist or at least care very much about what others think of you, you'll be less likely to take risks. Unless you are fully confident that you can garner success, you will find excuses to avoid a task you've previously failed at or never attempted before. If you're frustrated with an assignment, you may prefer to engage in something less frustrating. And if you're bored with your work, you might seek stimulation elsewhere.

Fear of failure is related to a fear of rejection. It comes from a belief that you are inadequate, and each failure therefore feels like a reminder about your lack of worth. No one likes to feel this way, so we try to prevent this situation from happening by shifting our focus to other safer ways to spend our time.

Procrastination may seem like a great strategy, and it's a survival mechanism. If there was a snake in your path you would be smart to avoid it, but that's also how your brain functions in the office. The trouble is that avoidance keeps you stuck in a perpetual pattern. You never overcome your fears this way. To truly get over such obstacles, you have to face your fears. That means taking risks and trying something even if success is not guaranteed because the path to growth is through learning from mistakes.

Even with the best of intentions, you can find yourself getting stuck, dragging your feet, and inadvertently watching deadlines creep closer and closer.

What You Can Learn from a Spider About Time Management

We all have busy and demanding lives. Our biggest challenge can be how to increase productivity while keeping our sanity. One of the best time management lessons comes from a children's book.

In *The Very Busy Spider*, Eric Carle writes about a spider incredibly focused on a singular task: spinning a web. Throughout the book, different animals approach the spider and ask whether she would like to have a fun experience with them. In each instance, the spider doesn't answer them and continues on. At the end of that busy day of spinning the web is complete and the spider is so tired, she has fallen asleep.[2]

From this book, there are three lessons you can learn to help your productivity. First, you need to focus on one task at a time and make it your most important job. Work that only you can do demands your primary attention. Everything else can be delegated or outsourced.

Second, expect constant distractions and plan accordingly. When you have a plan to handle distractions, you will be more productive. Turn off devices. Let coworkers or family members and friends know that you are unavailable for calls, conversations, and hanging out until you finish your project.

Third, get good at estimating task length. If you're focused on a single project, ask yourself how long it will realistically take. You may just focus on a task that is a portion of the larger project. How much time do you have, and what can you achieve during that time? If need be, work with a timer to keep you focused and ensure you're taking breaks throughout the day. One such timer is the Pomodoro Technique, which reminds you to take 5-minute breaks after each 25-minute period of work.[3] If you follow these three tips, you too will be able to pull off your to-do list productively and efficiently.

Too many tabs open on a computer or too many applications open on the phone make the system run slowly. Imagine what it does to you when you have too many things you are trying to accomplish at once. To avoid being overwhelmed, dilute your to-do list. Prioritize the jobs that will have the most impact if you get them done first: the most critical tasks. Eliminate distractions. Instead of multitasking, have a singular focus on one task at a time and you'll become masterfully effective. Like an elevator or an airplane, you have to know how much weight you can carry, and after that start turning things down.

Trish's Failure to Launch

Trish, an HR professional in a bustling tech company, was drowning in a sea of tasks. Her desk resembled a paperwork avalanche and her email inbox was an ever-expanding black hole. Trish was trapped in the cycle of procrastination, and through our coach-

---

TABLE 20.1 Prioritizating Effectively

- Focus on important and urgent tasks.
- Focus on tasks that only you can do.
- Delegate or outsource all remaining tasks.
- Expect distractions and plan accordingly.
- Work with a timer to stay mindful and take breaks.
- Focus on one thing at a time.

ing sessions I uncovered three primary reasons that drove her to postpone dealing with her overwhelming workload.

What any procrastinator will tell you is that the more you procrastinate, the more you procrastinate. In other words, work piles up when you're putting things off. The more it piles up, the more overwhelmed you feel by it, the more you put it off. The solution was clear: She needed to break up her workload into manageable chunks. We counted how many files she needed to get done, how long it takes her to complete one such file, and then calculated how many she can reasonably get done in a day, which led to the magic number of how many days she would need to get it all done. Simply having this plan in mind gave her enough relief to get started.

But there was more. The second reason Trish was stumped was that her workspace was a chaotic maze of scattered documents and sticky notes. Her lack of an efficient organizational system hindered her productivity. The remedy? Implementing a structured calendar.

I advised Trish to create a comprehensive calendar that accounted for all her responsibilities, not just meetings. By doing so she could identify free time slots and allocate them to essential HR tasks, including handling employee matters and conducting interviews. Only half-jokingly I told her, "You have to live religiously by the calendar. You are predetermining your destiny!"

The third reason for Trish's procrastination was that, simply stated, she wasn't excited about the tasks. She didn't like doing them, and then resentment would set in when she thought, "I'd rather be doing something else."

When you think negatively about a task as Trish did, not doing the task becomes the reward. But what is the consequence? It hangs over you. Trish described it as, "There's a sense of something on my back. I know I just need to get it done, but I'm getting further and further behind." To make matters worse, she would also think, "If I'm not able to get what I need done, maybe I'm not good enough." Clearly her thinking was getting in the way.

What was lacking for Trish was motivation, and that is exactly what she needed in order to get activated. To get there she needed to change her thoughts. Instead of having the temporary reward be avoidance of an unpleasant task (followed by negative emotions for having the work hanging over her), I asked her what it's costing her to delay the work. This helped her come up with alternative thoughts that made engaging in these tasks feel rewarding.

Trish realized that by doing the work when it came across her desk, she wouldn't have to feel anxious about the future. She wouldn't have the pressure of work piling up. She would get the weekend off rather than using that time to catch up on work. And she would feel more confident in herself.

Matt's Follow-Through Challenge

Sometimes, though, the issue isn't in getting started; it's in pushing through. Matt was someone who tended to over-promise and under-deliver. He came to see me because he wanted to increase his follow-through so he could move forward in his career.

When Matt showed up for our first meeting, his energy struck me immediately. He was charismatic, enthusiastic, and ambitious. Matt had big dreams of what he wanted to accomplish and how he wanted to contribute but had fallen short in his delivery, which led to him being fired from jobs time after time. While losing a job due to lack of productivity would be hard on anyone, it was especially hard on Matt because he felt stuck and unfulfilled. There was so much desire within him to be productive, yet he didn't know how to overcome this invisible hurdle.

The first thing that made a difference in Matt's productivity was the use of the app Rescuetime.[4] If you're not familiar with this tool, it tracks your online activity, thereby giving you insight and motivation to improve your performance. It does this by helping you decrease the time you spend on distractions and focus more on the essential aspects of your job. It provides one of the key ingredients in helping you be successful: accountability. And it does this by increasing your self-awareness.

This brings us to the second element for follow-through success: self-efficacy. When you believe you are capable, you are more likely to feel confident, take more risks, and achieve more. Your accomplishments will then continually increase your self-efficacy.

Conversely, when you lack a belief in your ability, you experience more self-doubt, use avoidance as a coping strategy to protect yourself from your projected failure and accomplish less. You then fall into the trap of believing that the reason you didn't achieve what you wanted to is that you weren't capable, when in truth it was because you didn't try.

Matt understood that by changing his belief in his ability, he would be able to get things done. His lack of follow-through stemmed, for the most part, from his insecurities and self-doubt. Once he was able to see his self-limiting belief as an obstacle and reshape it to align with his desired outcome, he became unstoppable.

The third and final nugget that drastically improved Matt's success was when he started valuing his effort, not just the outcome. Many of us get overwhelmed by all that we have to do. It can seem like our lists are never ending. The more expectations others have of us, the less we will get done and, of course, if we value outcomes and are not getting as much done as we would like, we can start to feel bad about ourselves.

When you invest time and energy into a task, sometimes it will flop, and other times it will work out well. When things don't go your way, you are put to the test. How do you talk to yourself? By appreciating your investment of resources, you are focusing on the journey, not just the destination.

This is also essential when a task is large and may require you to work on it for several days. Just because the entire mission isn't complete after one day doesn't mean you didn't get anything done. Be realistic in your expectations given the resources at your disposal. According to Matt, "Doing small tasks builds up the ability to do bigger tasks."

There's Always Tomorrow Today

If you find yourself struggling with procrastination, work to increase your personal competency skills, especially emotional management. One way of managing difficult emotions related to a task is by forgiving yourself. Researchers found that when students forgave themselves after procrastinating on studying for a first exam, their procrastination subsequently went down when they needed to prepare for a second exam. The reason these students cited for this shift was that self-forgiveness helped them to regulate their negative emotions.[5]

In every situation, we can find positive and negative aspects. Tasks on the job are no exception. The next time you are feeling negative about a task, ask yourself what aspect of that task is positive. If you lack confidence in performing well on this task, consider what tasks you've worked on in the past that were similar and on which you did well.

You might also think about what positive outcomes may come from completing this task. By shifting your perspective from a negative to a more positive aspect, you can bypass procrastination and get to work.

You might be wondering, "If I've struggled with procrastination my entire life, will it take me another lifetime to make these changes?" The answer is no. Most people believe that it takes about 21 days to create new habits. From my experience this is usually true for small habits, especially habits of mind (i.e., self-efficacy beliefs), but for behavioral change it can take longer.

The good news is that while it may take longer than three weeks, it doesn't have to take a lifetime. Matt, who had struggled with a lack of follow-through for over three decades, was able to become productive in just under three months.

So if launching or lack of follow-through are what you struggle with, take note, as you too can have a renewed experience, feel better about yourself, and do so in about 90 days.

It is too easy to run away from aspects of work deemed unpleasant, too challenging, or boring. But if you want to be productive and give yourself a real chance to succeed, you need to implement emotional management skills and embrace the task.

Remember, people procrastinate for different reasons, and each of them needs to be addressed individually. For feeling overwhelmed, there's chunking. For disorganization, there's calendaring. For lack of motivation, there's refocusing on the benefit of doing the work now so you can have the luxury of free time later.

For you to easily remember the three aspects you need to incorporate into your routine to increase follow up, think ABC:

TABLE 20.2 **Increasing Your Follow-Through**

- Track your activity or have someone keep you accountable.
- Work to increase self-efficacy and eliminate insecurities and self-doubt.
- Value your effort, not just the outcome.
- Have realistic expectations. Just because the task isn't completely done doesn't mean you didn't get anything done.
- Forgive yourself for any mistakes you make.
- Identify the positive aspects of tasks, even when they feel negative.
- If you lack confidence to perform a task, consider its similarities to tasks that you were able to do in the past.
- Identify the positives that would come from completing this task.
- List the risks you might be taking to overcome the problem and the prices you'll continue to pay if you don't achieve your goal.

---

1. **Accountability:** Find an accountability system that keeps track of your activity and sustains your motivation to improve with continual feedback.

2. **Belief:** Work on your belief in yourself to make your self-fulfilling prophecy a positive rather than a negative one.

3. **Credit:** Give yourself credit for your efforts, not just your outcomes. With this compassionate approach, you will build up your confidence, get more done in less time, and feel good about your accomplishments.

PERFECT ATTENTION

One of the most significant ways we lose time is when we are distracted. It's easier than ever in today's workplace to become distracted from essential tasks we intend to accomplish.

We have computers, phones, meetings, papers, people, and objects all around us. Emails stream in constantly. Texts and calls come in when we least expect them. Just when you get into the groove of your work, something takes your attention offline.

To be excellent at work you have to have perfect attention. If you were the CEO of the company, you could make executive decisions about what you say "yes" and "no" to. Similarly, you are the CEO of yourself. You need to make executive decisions about how to manage your time, and one of the best ways to increase engagement is by decreasing distractions.

Decide to turn off notifications and check your emails, voice-mails, and texts during breaks rather than throughout the day. Decide to avoid small talk with those around you so you can focus on your work. Decide to spend your time on your most important tasks while your energy is high so you don't have to cram and stress over your to-do list once you're exhausted and coming up on a deadline.

Making these types of decisions comes from a place of empowerment. And while eliminating distractions can help anyone be more efficient at work, it is especially crucial for those who have less flexibility of time.

An interesting phenomenon happens when you have less time but more purpose. Rather than feeling overwhelmed and stressed, you become focused and get more done in the same timeframe.

This phenomenon is particularly evident among working mothers. Their efficiency tends to soar because they are acutely aware of the strict cut-off time when they must leave the office. With a clear sense of purpose, they zero in on their priorities. They become more assertive about not taking on large projects or shouldering their colleagues' work. These mothers approach their tasks as if there's a daily deadline looming. There's no room for procrastination or distraction. They have a commitment, whether it's picking up their child or tending to their child's care-giver, and they manage their dual responsibilities in both their professional and personal lives with remarkable dedication.

Consider what purpose awaits you outside of the office. If you don't have a family, perhaps schedule an exercise class or a dinner date with a friend or engage in a leisure activity after work. Knowing that you have a definite cut-off time will help you focus on your work and enjoy the benefits of increased work-life balance.

Perfect attention results from eliminating distractions and creating boundaries around your time. Be intentional about how you engage in the workplace because this will determine

---

TABLE 20.3 **Perfecting Your Attention**

- Decrease distractions.
  - Turn off notifications.
  - Check messages during breaks.
  - Avoid small talk.
- Find purpose outside the office and create a hard cut-off time to leave work.
- Protect your time and say no to taking on projects you can't realistically afford to take on.

not only how quickly you finish your work but how much time you have to engage in more personal matters.

CONCLUSION

Effective time management hinges on three fundamental components.

First, it involves the art of prioritization—identifying and concentrating on your most crucial tasks one by one.

Second, it thrives on fostering engagement in your work. Instead of procrastinating or avoiding daunting challenges, confront them directly. Embrace risks and commit to completing tasks. Cultivate self-compassion and work diligently to boost your self-assurance.

Third, it centers on focusing your attention and creating an environment that nurtures productivity. This can be achieved by eliminating distractions, safeguarding your time, and establishing a clear boundary between work and personal life. These strategies serve to enhance your focus and elevate your overall efficiency.

Exercise for Step 3

To build on what you have done so far and take the next appropriate action, follow these three steps to increase your engagement:

Step 1: Now that you are clear on your needs (step 1) and feel empowered (step 2), it's time to find ways to increase engagement. Fill out the table below.

- Column 1: List your needs.

- Column 2: Specify the job resources you require (e.g., mentoring, increased control, task variety, communication, fairness, value congruence, feedback, opportunities for learning and development, career perspective) to align with your needs.

- Column 3: Outline strategies to boost optimal engagement.

- Column 4: Highlight methods for enhancing productivity.

This will serve to organize your thoughts and clarify your message before you ask for what you want.

Step 2: Communicate to your manager about the information in the table above clearly and concisely utilizing the skills you learned about assertiveness in chapter 9.

Step 3: Elicit feedback for your contributions. Feedback allows for both professional growth and a feeling that the work you are doing is meaningful, and this knowledge increases engagement. In other words, it's a strategic approach to continuous development and career success.

Needs	Job Resources	Ways to Increase Engagement	Ways to Improve Productivity

Efficacy

When you lack belief in your ability, you are more at risk for burning out, especially if your efficacy has been stripped away by work conditions. On the flip side, high self-efficacy correlates with engagement and follow-through.

According to Albert Bandura, a psychologist who wrote a lot about the construct of self-efficacy, your beliefs shape your expectations and affect your goal-setting, the amount of effort you put into a goal, and how persistently you cope with obstacles when pursuing that goal.[1]

In the next few chapters we will delve into the nature of three types of efficacy spirals. The first type is a *downward spiral*, as already described in chapter 19. The opposite, of course, is an *upward spiral*, in which you experience success in place of failure. The final spiral is what is known as a *self-correcting spiral*. By examining how these spirals work and how your thinking and performance are intertwined, you can learn how to take back your power.

CHAPTER 21

Self-Efficacy Spirals

In our busy and demanding world, we seek to find ways to become more efficient (get more done in less time) and effective (focus on activities that yield the greatest outcomes). While we know about efficiency and effectiveness, a third concept to consider is *efficacy*. It can make or break your success because it affects the tool you need most to help you move ahead: your mind.

While we've already mentioned that downward spirals are associated with failure and upward spirals are associated with success, we need to understand the basic tenets of these mechanisms. In the psychological literature, these phenomena are called "self-efficacy spirals." The reason there is a relationship between efficacy beliefs and success or failure is that self-efficacy and performance are interdependent (figure 21.1). The more you believe in your ability, the more likely you will pursue a task. The more successful you are in accomplishing a task, the more you will believe in your ability to do so in the future.

When your self-efficacy beliefs align with your effort levels, you may find yourself in one of two scenarios: an upward or a downward spiral. But there's also the possibility of encountering a self-correcting spiral, where initially, your performance and self-efficacy run in tandem, but then one of them shifts direction. How does this happen?

FIGURE 21.1 The efficacy–performance relationship.

Imagine you attempt to write code, but you don't get the results you want. You try again and again, but disappointment follows each attempt. If you expected your knowledge and efforts to translate into success and they don't, this may affect your belief in your ability to get the project off the ground. You may then procrastinate working on it or just give up. But perhaps after a cooling-off period, you review your steps, realize your mistake, and take a more successful approach. Your self-efficacy just increased, so you sit back down and try again, hence increasing your performance (figure 21.2).

The same situation can happen in reverse order (figure 21.3). You attempt your code and find that it works time and time again. This builds up your self-efficacy but can lead you to become overly confident and complacent. You decide that since you're so good at what you do, you don't have to try so hard. You become less motivated to figure out what is leading to your continued success. The result over the next succession of tasks reflects this change in effort and ends up leading to some failure

FIGURE 21.2   Self-Correcting Upward Spirals. *Sources*: Masuch, "Vicious Cycles in Organizations"; Karl E. Weick, *The Social Psychology of Organizing* (2nd ed.) (Reading, MA: Addison-Wesley, 1979).

as you experience a ceiling effect. Once again, your self-efficacy decreases, as does your performance.

The name of the game is to understand the cause-and-effect nature of task performance. When you recognize why your efforts lead to either success or failure, by keeping your finger on the pulse, you are increasing your chances of future successes. Otherwise, you are at risk of becoming overconfident. Therefore, one purpose of the self-correcting spiral is to promote learning, which keeps you moving in a vertical direction to achieve greater success over time.[1] Also, if after a chain of successes you become complacent, it helps turn that complacency into a downward spiral that keeps you in check.

FIGURE 21.3 Self-Correcting Downward Spirals. *Sources*: Masuch, "Vicious Cycles in Organizations"; Karl E. Weick, *The Social Psychology of Organizing* (2nd ed.) (Reading, MA: Addison-Wesley, 1979).

CONCLUSION

Your beliefs can affect your success and failure rates. When your efforts yield outcomes, you can either enter into an upward spiral in the wake of success or descend into a downward spiral following a failure. A self-correcting spiral can flip the direction of your efficacy such as when you become complacent after attaining success or when you learn from your mistakes after a failure. Be mindful of your beliefs and keep your attention in your work sharp.

CHAPTER 22

How Spirals Get Started

To stop or reverse a downward spiral, we first have to understand what constitutes a spiral, what gets spirals started, and what keeps them going.

Self-efficacy spirals are influenced by certain rules and factors that shape their dynamics:

1. *Minimum of three tasks*: To initiate a self-efficacy spiral, it's typically required that you have attempted at least three different tasks or challenges. This is because self-efficacy beliefs tend to evolve and solidify over multiple experiences rather than a single instance. After three attempts, patterns in your self-efficacy beliefs may start to become evident.

2. *Independence from success or failure*: Self-efficacy spirals are not contingent solely on whether you succeed or fail in a task. Instead, they are more related to how you interpret and respond to these outcomes. Whether you achieve success or face failure, it's your perception of these outcomes and the subsequent actions you take that influence the direction of the spiral.

3. *Learning from mistakes*: The optimal path within self-efficacy spirals involves learning from your

mistakes. Regardless of whether you initially succeed or fail, the ability to reflect on your performance, identify areas for improvement, and adjust your approach is essential. By learning and adapting from your experiences, you can drive your self-efficacy beliefs in a positive direction.[1]

Factors contributing to the formation and direction of self-efficacy spirals include:

1. *Feedback*: The feedback you receive from your attempts at tasks plays a significant role. Positive feedback, such as recognition for your accomplishments, can boost your self-efficacy. Conversely, negative feedback, if interpreted constructively, can also contribute to an upward spiral by motivating you to improve.

2. *Task uncertainty and complexity*: The nature of the tasks you undertake matters. Tasks characterized by high uncertainty and complexity can influence self-efficacy more profoundly. Facing such challenges can either lead to increased confidence if you conquer them or decreased confidence if you struggle. Task difficulty is a key driver of the spiral's direction.

3. *Task experience*: Your cumulative experience with various tasks also influences self-efficacy. The more exposure you have to different types of challenges, the more opportunities you have to shape your beliefs. Positive experiences can reinforce your self-efficacy whereas repeated negative experiences may erode it.

Some of these factors were discussed in chapter 19, but to better understand their contribution to a spiral, let's break them down.

FEEDBACK

Feedback is a necessary element for continued success or for preventing a downward spiral. It requires us to look at what we have done, whether or not it is working, and why. In a traditional work context, "feedback" refers to information received from a manager or supervisor whose job it is to examine your work and share their expertise and knowledge about your performance. To be effective, feedback needs to be accurate, timely, and specifically address the cause-and-effect nature of your performance. Feedback that misses the mark on any of these three factors is ineffective and can start a spiral.

If you work on tasks, especially challenging ones where you have less knowledge or experience, it is crucial for you to receive effective feedback. Assert your needs and focus on clear communication between you and your boss.

TASK UNCERTAINTY AND COMPLEXITY

When you are trying out a task that is completely new to you, your boss, or your organization, or even the person to whom you report will not know the causal relationship of your performance to the outcome.

This ignorance means you are unlikely to receive the feedback you need. Similarly, when tasks are complex, there could be more than one cause-and-effect factor, which translates into less clarity and possible confusion. The less you understand about what leads to success, the higher your chances of failure and the greater the likelihood of a spiral starting.

If you are working on an original project, keep your expectations realistic. Expect to ride the wave of self-efficacy spirals and know that they are there to promote your long-term learning. Rather than becoming attached to your immediate results, stay focused on the big picture and prepare yourself for turbulence. If, however, your task is new only to you but has been done before, consider consulting with someone who has experience with it, even if it means finding a mentor outside your place of work.

TASK EXPERIENCE

When experience is low, if you are successful in your attempt, you may make mistaken attributions for your success. This misinformation can lead you to take a wrong turn or, as mentioned earlier, to become overconfident, which can start a spiral. During this early period, the focus is on increased learning. You are learning about causality, what leads to success, what leads to failure, and why these relationships exist. Note that your self-efficacy is strongly affected by initial successes or failures. So the more you fail initially, for example, the weaker your self-efficacy beliefs and the lower you can expect your performance to be. With this in mind, avoid the trap of being too quickly influenced by early results. Focus instead on garnering more experience on a given task to prevent a negative spiral from starting.

CONCLUSION

After attempting a task at least three times, you might enter a downward spiral if you meet any of these conditions: You receive inaccurate, untimely, or unspecific feedback; you are uncertain about the cause-and-effect nature of a task, or the task is complex; or you lack experience related to the task at hand. The opposite of these conditions can contribute to an upward spiral. Given this knowledge, you can be mindful of how to handle yourself at work and what to ask for to perform to the best of your abilities. By focusing on learning rather than on the outcome, you can increase your overall performance over time.

CHAPTER 23

What Keeps Spirals Going

Four factors keep spirals going: attributions, automatic information processing, emotional arousal, and expectations and labels.[1]

ATTRIBUTIONS

Just as accurate feedback is important, proper attributions (or the causality you assign to your task performance) are essential. Proper attributions can help correct behaviors when you are making errors. Errors in attribution can lead to more mistakes.

Different attribution errors affect performance. If you attribute failures or successes to yourself, that is an internal attribution. While at times you might contribute to a task's failure, its failure does not necessarily mean you alone are at fault. Often there are external factors that contribute to a lack of success. Alternatively, you might attribute all the blame to external factors and not take any responsibility for mistakes you have made. This is an attempt to conserve your self-efficacy because when faced with failure, if you attribute the failure to yourself, you will become anxious.

A second attribution error relates to stability. Because spirals occur after three or more consecutively stable wins or losses, you are likely to attribute the win or loss to a stable factor such as your ability. When you've failed multiple times in a row and you associate that failure with your inability, this can lead to discouragement. Conversely, when you attribute the win or loss to instability with statements like "I didn't invest adequate effort in this," the loss is less likely to decrease your self-efficacy. Adopt Thomas Edison's approach. After experiencing more failures than most people you'll likely ever meet, Edison said, "'I have not failed. I've just found 10,000 ways that won't work.'"[2]

Lastly, when you inaccurately attribute your performance to the degree of control you have over the situations, you are making a controllability attribution error. It is important to understand that even in situations where you may have limited control over certain aspects of a process or outcome, there are often elements within your sphere of influence that can be harnessed. For instance, when you experience anxiety, if you focus on regulating your breathing, you can change your state even in the face of an event that feels scary and is out of your control. It is when you believe you have no control that you end up feeling frustrated, anxious, or helpless and continue a downward spiral.

When you attribute your success or failure to factors that are internal, stable, and over which you lack control, you are more certain to remain in a spiral. Consider what external, unstable, and controllable factors may have contributed to your performance and take these into account to get the full story of what's transpired.

AUTOMATIC INFORMATION PROCESSING

When your performance outcomes repeat, your brain is more likely to process information associated with those outcomes automatically. This automated processing is quicker and tends to be more superficial. For instance, organizations that year after year yield success often stop analyzing what led to their outcomes. Instead they focus on maintaining stability, and over time, they start to decline due to the belief that they are invulnerable.

Blockbuster was a sensational business, renting the latest releases of movies to customers from their many brick-and-mortar locations. But as consumer needs began to change and people wanted digital access to media or to have films shipped to them for greater convenience, Blockbuster fell behind the curve. Only six years after Netflix launched its services did Blockbuster begin to test-drive the new model, but by then they had missed the boat.

Formerly thriving companies such as Kodak, Nokia, Black-Berry, Toys "R" Us, and Sears offer valuable lessons underscoring the significance of consistently seeking comprehensive feedback even in the midst of success. In an ever-evolving landscape, consumer preferences evolve, rendering strategies that once led to triumph potentially obsolete. What propels success today may fall short of meeting future demands; the need for adaptability and ongoing feedback to remain competitive and relevant is perpetual. Don't let what happened to these companies happen to you. Stay vigilant and curious.

EMOTIONAL AROUSAL

We are emotional beings, and our experience at work is no exception. Our performance affects how we feel, and how we feel can impact our performance. We've already mentioned the importance of attributions (the meanings we give to our results). The next step in the chain is to consider how the way that we think affects how we feel at work. When we make mistaken attributions that are internal, stable, and uncontrollable, we are more likely to feel a sense of despair, which will negatively affect our efficacy and thus our performance.

If you're feeling discouraged or frustrated, your negative mood may lead you to interpret information through a more negative lens associated with low self-efficacy. Similarly, heightened fear can interfere with your performance. When emotional arousal is high, spirals become more prominent.

Be mindful of your mood. Staying in the task with negativity does you no good. When you feel negative, either take time out to recalibrate or reframe your anxiety as "excitement" to shift the energy and your potential downward spiral.

EXPECTATIONS AND LABELS

We don't rise to the level of our expectations,
we fall to the level of our training.
ARCHILOCHOS

The Pygmalion effect is when your expectations become your reality.[3] High expectations lead to high performance, while low expectations lead to poor performance. This is not only true of your expectations of yourself; other people's expectations of your performance have just as much of an impact. When you have a stable outcome over time, you may start adopting a label for yourself as a "winner" or a "loser."

It's crucial to emphasize that your mindset and effort are the true drivers of success. Whether you achieve or fall short of a particular goal is secondary. What truly matters is your commitment to continuous learning, as this signifies genuine progress.

Avoid limiting self-labels, as outcomes don't define your identity; your relentless efforts do.

CONCLUSION

Once a self-efficacy spiral starts, it's essential to understand what keeps it going so that you can intervene correctly. To this end, you must correctly attribute what leads to success and failure. Avoid processing information on autopilot and, instead, stay analytically minded. Be conscious of how your mood affects your performance. Pay attention to performance-related expectations. Above all, resist the urge to label yourself based solely on outcomes; remember that your efforts and the lessons learned from them define your journey.

CHAPTER 24

How to Stop a Downward Spiral

While it may be easier to avoid a spiral than to stop or change it, there are two ways to end a spiral. These techniques are both cognitive and behavioral.

REDEFINING SUCCESS AND FAILURE

One of the main reasons we experience lowered self-efficacy is that we are attached to the idea of success as a reflection of our ability. Researchers suggest that "success is not based on the outcome, but it comes from the information gained via the task attempt."[1] By redefining your success as what you've learned as opposed to what you've accomplished, you can stop a downward spiral and help preserve your self-efficacy. When you define success in this way, you fail only if you do not learn. Even when you obtain the results you set out to get, if you do not learn something new and simply rely on what made you successful in the past, you are not truly successful by this new definition.

Given what we know about what leads to downward spirals and what keeps them going, seeing your work as opportunities to experiment, attain high-quality feedback, reduce arousal, and decrease automatic processing of information can help to stop and even prevent the spiral.

SMALL WINS AND LOSSES

As mentioned earlier, one of the factors that can prompt a spiral to start is task complexity. When the tasks you are going after are too big, focus your efforts on small chunks. Break tasks down to simplify your mission. Doing so will reduce the risk of massive failures, provide more opportunities for learning, and help you build up your self-efficacy when you have small wins. Besides, this will have a positive effect on your emotional arousal.

While James Watson and Francis Crick worked on discovering the structure of DNA, which eventually led to them being awarded the Nobel Prize in Physiology or Medicine 1962, they observed that their attitude largely contributed to their progress. This was later called the "Progress Principle."[2] That is, when you make progress in meaningful work (small wins), you feel most accomplished.

Your progress might feel insignificant in comparison to the total project and what needs to get done. To change your view of it, keep a list of your small wins so you can reflect back on them and see how the list has grown over time. By keeping each small victory in perspective with your total wins, you will see how you are making meaningful progress.

CONCLUSION

As we've already seen, spirals can be corrected. So, if you find yourself in a downward spiral, don't despair. There are effective measures you can take to stop its descent. Begin by redefining your perception of success and failure, thereby allowing for a more balanced and constructive perspective. Additionally, breaking down complex tasks into manageable components can prevent failures from becoming insurmountable obstacles. Finally, maintain a record of your small victories to serve as a constant reminder of your numerous accomplishments. When you do so, work regains its intrinsic meaning and purpose.

Exercise for Step 4

Individuals who have successful experiences and who attribute those successes to themselves have higher self-efficacy. Below, list your past successes that resulted from your efforts.

_____

_____

_____

_____

_____

_____

_____

PART III

Passive Presence

Energy

Every day, as you come across life's challenges, tasks, and responsibilities, you exert energy. When you expend energy without replenishing it, you rapidly burn out.

As discussed in chapter 20, the concept of prioritization isn't limited to the workplace alone. It extends to all facets of your life, including your personal sphere.

One of the biggest hurdles busy professionals point to when it comes to taking care of themselves is a lack of time. In this section we will tackle time management as it relates to self-care.

Time, however, is rarely the real reason why we don't prioritize ourselves. Usually, there are mindset obstacles. In chapter 25, I will show you how to overcome these before you dive into your self-care practices.

Once your thinking aligns with your desire to recharge, you will need to find what self-care practices work best for you. In chapter 26, I will delve into ways to protect and recover your energy. If you notice that even when you are taking measures to fill up your energy tank, you are just not feeling energized enough, don't worry. To address this, I will discuss recovery strategies customized to your personality.

Part of managing your energy is about creating healthy boundaries. In chapter 27, I will share with you the price that having poor boundaries can have on you. I will debunk the myths you might hold that prevent you from having better boundaries and provide you with some suggestions on changes you can make.

Finally, chapter 28 focuses on transitioning out of work in ways that help you create balance, increase your happiness, and energize you to continue doing your job effectively.

CHAPTER 25

Mindset Obstacles to Self-Care

While the concept of incorporating self-care into your life isn't groundbreaking, the fact that many individuals struggle to integrate it into their routines suggests there's more to explore. For some, prioritizing self-care can be an uphill battle, often due to the perception that their needs hold less significance than those of others. This internal struggle can manifest as feelings of guilt whenever they do something for themselves, indicating a deep-rooted mindset issue. The journey from self-sacrifice to self-nourishment begins with addressing this mindset.

Perhaps you've taken pride in your role as a constant care-taker, finding purpose in providing for others. While there's nothing inherently wrong with this altruistic approach, problems arise when it becomes one-sided and you neglect your own needs. Do acts of self-care genuinely make you uncomfortable or conflicted? If so, it's crucial to explore and understand this internal conflict to reshape your feelings toward self-care.

In my work with many individuals who've experienced burn-out, a common thread is their failure to prioritize self-care adequately. Take Shawna, for instance, a client who grappled with the belief that any self-nourishment, even mundane activities like cleaning her closet, felt extravagant and selfish. Shawna's relentless commitment to caring for others mirrored the role of a martyr, leaving her perpetually feeling insufficient and unjustifiably apologetic for her own needs.

If you find yourself in a situation similar to Shawna's, where even a well-crafted self-care plan and a newfound appreciation for its importance aren't enough to break the cycle, it's vital to address the underlying beliefs that have led to this predicament. Start by identifying the specific beliefs that obstruct your engagement in self-care and recognize that they no longer serve your well-being. To transform your behavior, you must first transform your beliefs. One highly effective approach to achieve this transformation is through affirmations or mantras. With your limiting beliefs in mind, craft alternative beliefs that align with the practice of regular self-care. Observe individuals who prioritize self-care and consider the beliefs that empower them to do so.

Shawna recalled listening to other moms mention that they went out and bought a camera. This camera, however, was not for their kids. It was not for taking pictures of the family. It was to record their own tennis match. This blew Shawna's mind because, as she said, "That's never something I would do." But when she was able to think about the kinds of beliefs these moms must have, she said, "Well, they must really believe that they're important." As a result, she was able to come up with her own mantra which was, "I am worth it." Shawna's mantra can be a mantra for anyone who struggles with prioritizing themselves.

You may not believe that mantra at first. The second step is to practice saying it until you get to a place where it feels true. Ask yourself, "How much do I currently believe my mantra on a scale of 0 to 100 (if 0 is 'not at all' and 100 is 'absolutely true')?" Shawna started out believing the mantra only 30 percent, but as she practiced it day in and day out, her belief significantly changed.

> **TABLE 25.1 Overcoming Mindset Obstacles to Self-Care**
>
> - *Prioritize self-care*: Recognize that caring for yourself enables you to better care for others.
> - *Identify limiting beliefs*: Understand the root causes of self-doubt and negative beliefs about self-worth.
>
> **Self-Reflection:**
> - *Assess your belief*: On a scale of 0 to 100, how strongly do you believe in your worthiness of self-care? (0 = not at all, 100 = completely)
> - *Practice self-affirmation*: Repeat the mantra "I am worthy of self-care" daily to reinforce positive beliefs.
> - *Track your progress*: Weekly, reassess your belief in your worthiness and note any shifts.
>
> **Embracing Self-Care:**
> - *Align actions with beliefs*: Once you believe in your worthiness, implement self-care strategies that align with your values and goals.

Once your beliefs undergo this pivotal shift, it's time for the third step: devising a repertoire of self-care activities to integrate into your life. Reflect on activities that genuinely bring you joy and replenish your spirit. For instance, if dancing resonates with you, consider joining a dance class. If exercise invigorates your body and mind, explore your preferences—whether it's outdoor jogging or gym workouts. Mindfulness practices, such as meditation, offer an excellent avenue for relaxation and have been scientifically proven to yield various benefits.[1] Don't forget to prioritize physical relaxation, perhaps scheduling monthly massages or establishing a weekly ritual of unwinding in a soothing bath. The goal is to identify activities that help you manage stress effectively, thereby enabling you to provide better support to others while safeguarding yourself against burnout.

CONCLUSION

Self-care is essential to prevent burnout, but a negative mind-set can get in the way. To overcome this obstacle, start by identifying your limiting beliefs. Create mantras that help you prioritize yourself and practice them until they feel true. Once you believe you are worth it, you will easily align your behaviors with your newfound belief and start taking proper care of yourself.

CHAPTER 26

Managing Your Energy

Once you're on board with the belief that self-care is nonnegotiable, the next obstacle on your path might be finding the time to incorporate it into your day. It's easy to get caught in a catch-22. Sometimes, when you have a lot on your plate, you might think you don't have time for yourself. You work hard to push through and get things done. But when you don't take care of yourself in the process, you might notice that you enjoy the work you are doing less, that you have less energy, and that you are less efficient in getting it done. The formula for success is scheduling your self-care and then everything else around it.

Create a "red velvet rope policy" around your time, treating yourself like a VIP. This shift in perception underscores the true importance of attending to your needs before anything else. If you're an entrepreneur, seizing control of your schedule becomes more feasible. Identify moments during the day to engage in workouts, as motivation tends to wane after extended work hours. For employees, consider negotiating for an extended lunch break to accommodate exercise or arrange for occasional remote workdays. Collaborating with a coworker as an accountability partner can be motivating, especially for after-work gym sessions. Additionally, committing to specific days and times for fitness classes enhances your chances of consistent attendance.

Equally important is avoiding overscheduling. One practical approach is to assess your future availability before committing to social engagements. If you foresee a continued high level of busyness next month, refrain from scheduling yourself to future events. While committing to an engagement usually means feeling obligated to attend when the date arrives, excessive commitments can lead to either reluctant attendance or last-minute cancellations. Strive for realistic expectations regarding your capacity within the confines of your available time.

One of the biggest mistakes we make is underestimating how long tasks take. I used to do this all the time. I would have three plates spinning at once with the overly optimistic notion that I could prevent them from crashing down. When you take on too much, you stress yourself out and are always on the run. By taking on less, I learned that I could be on time or even early to a meeting with someone and that extra time gives me breathing room, especially when the unexpected happens. If there is traffic, if parking spots are limited, or if I want some time to gather my thoughts before I meet with a friend or colleague, having a few extra moments can make a big difference in how I present myself. Now, I ask myself how long it might take to get somewhere or complete a task and then double my estimation to leave additional time for the unexpected.

When you make self-care a top priority, you guarantee that you'll allocate time for it. Maintaining a sense of realism about your future commitments ensures that you won't overextend yourself. Allowing for generous time margins around your engagements helps reduce potential stress.

RECOVERING YOUR ENERGY

Scheduling your self-care practices is a great way to have time carved out to re-energize. Now you just have to incorporate the types of activities that will help you recover your energy, especially if you're starting from a place of burnout.

Every car has a gauge that tells you when it is low on gas. To continue driving it, you have to fill up the tank. Similarly, you need to gauge your energy level and find ways to refuel, especially when you feel yourself dragging.

Some people seek out instant energy boosts in the form of sugar, nicotine, or caffeine, while others look for rapid relaxation and stress relief with options such as alcohol, marijuana, or benzodiazepines. These methods can calm your nerves and allow your brain to slow down and take a break from worrying thoughts.

The problem with these approaches is that they are short-lived. Not only will they not sustain energy levels for long, but you will experience a crash, requiring you to refuel over and over again. They don't dramatically change your pattern, either. They are quick fixes that provide momentary relief. But when you wake up tomorrow, you'll be back in the same boat.

Managing emotions is much easier to do when you routinely take time to destress. Creating healthy habits is a great way to recover from daily events and prevent becoming overwhelmed. Structure these 10 self-care practices into your week and then find a way to fit the rest of your world around them.

1. *Sleep.* Research has shown the implications of sleep on our mood,[1] not to mention our motivation and ability to focus. Most people require eight hours on average. Know your body's requirement and get to

bed on time rather than wasting time in the evening
mindlessly checking your social media accounts or
email or flipping through television stations. If need
be, set an alarm to remind you to start winding
down your activities and get into bed.

2. *Physical activity.* We spend many of our waking hours
   sitting in transit, at our jobs, or in front of a screen.
   Our bodies start to hurt when we don't move
   enough. Build in time each day to stretch and take
   walks. Several times per week, find time to exercise
   your muscles, build up strength, and increase flexibility. Moving your body helps exert energy and provides you a physical outlet to release anxiety and
   stress. It gets you out of the future and into the
   present.

3. *Nutrition.* When we are busy, we sometimes forget to
   eat. This can mean that we fall out of a scheduled
   routine and eat later than usual or skip meals altogether and then notice a shortage of energy or a
   headache coming on. Alternatively, we might over-
   eat, eat out of convenience, or eat to avoid feeling an
   unpleasant emotion. Food is your fuel. You need to
   make good choices, plan your meals, and use food
   appropriately as nourishment.

4. *Water.* In addition to minding your food intake, you
   need to hydrate your body with plenty of water
   throughout the day. Many of the popular beverages
   people consume, particularly coffee, can be dehy-
   drating. Even when you aren't physically active or
   exposed to the blistering sun, you lose liquids sitting
   in air-conditioned or heated environments. You also

wake up dehydrated each morning after hours of sleep. That's why it's important to drink water first thing each day as well as throughout the day and to minimize substances that contain caffeine, sugar, or other additives. Water helps with digestion and can keep you working at a more optimal level.

5. *Meditation.* Meditation has several uses. You can get into a routine of daily meditation, which acts as a vitamin to protect your immune system. You can also take a timeout when you're stressed and meditate for a few minutes as a way to get back to center. In this way, meditation serves as a tool for emotional regulation as it slows down your reaction time. It's an opportunity to sit quietly, train the mind to let go of worries, stressors, and plans, and be present. Meditation allows you to tune in to your body and notice any tension or pain. It's a time to focus on breathing, relaxing, and just being without doing.

6. *Grounding.* Grounding techniques help anchor us back to the present moment, reconnecting us with our bodies and the environment around us. By practicing grounding regularly, you can reduce stress, improve focus, and enhance your overall well-being. Simple techniques like feeling your feet on the floor, touching different textures, or describing objects in your immediate surroundings can quickly bring you back to center.

7. *Nature.* Spending time in nature is a very grounding experience, which can help regulate anxiety and fear states. It's an opportunity to breathe fresh air, to reconnect to your roots, and to relax without the

bustling noises of modern society. Moreover, exposure to sunlight is paramount for absorbing essential vitamin D, which, when lacking, can heighten the risk of depression, particularly during the winter months; this is yet another incentive to embrace the outdoors.[2] In addition, early-day exposure to sunlight plays a pivotal role in regulating the circadian rhythm, enhancing your overall sleep quality, mood, and productivity.

8. *Journaling*. A habit that produces a more positive mindset is gratitude journaling. Just ask yourself what in your life you are grateful for. The answers can be as simple as the sun shining, your partner's smile that greeted you on awakening, or even a good night's sleep. Furthermore, researchers have found that 20 minutes of daily writing about positive emotions helps reduce stress and anxiety.[3] By spending time writing about what's going well, you can improve your mood and build resilience to face future challenges. Once you've written about your day, you can go back and review your writing through a different lens. This helps you identify thinking traps, such as mind reading, overgeneralization, or prediction, and reframe your thoughts so they are more helpful to you.

9. *Breathing*. Breathing is an essential function for survival, yet it often becomes shallow in our daily lives. It's beneficial to incorporate mindful deep breathing into your routine, whether during meditation or moments of stress. Deep breaths facilitate the flow of energy throughout your body and help

regulate your emotions. Being mindful of your bodily sensations can make you more attuned to instances when you unconsciously hold your breath. Practicing breath awareness serves as a gentle reminder to release any tension and return to a calm state.

10. *Social support.* Because humans are wired for connection, when you share your feelings tactfully with others, you feel happier. Social support is considered not only a positive experience but a coping strategy that helps you get through difficult times. The alternative is isolation, which leads to depression and loneliness. Ask for help when you need it. Getting support from others will create bonds and help you achieve more of your goals.

To top it off, practice the "Taking Down the Flame" technique by Donna Eden to ground your energy. You can find a demonstration of this exercise on www.BurnoutToResilience.com.

CUSTOMIZED RECOVERY STRATEGY

Stress is about perception. What might be stressful to one person may not affect someone else at all or may lead to entirely different results in a third individual. When considering recovery strategies, you need to keep individual differences in mind and, in particular, how you obtain your energy.

In chapter 18 we talked about how introverts turn inward to recharge because being around other people takes a toll on their energy levels. Extroverts, on the other hand, need to be around others to restore their energy. Given the distinct differences between introverts and extroverts, it's essential to implement recovery strategies that fit your personality type.

Typically, introverts benefit from being alone or with one other person. Coping strategies that can help introverts recover their energy include taking a long walk, journaling, or exercising. These are all forms of grounding that anchor frantic energy and release stress from the mind and body.

Introverts also thrive when they minimize stimulation in their environment. This can involve proactive measures in various aspects of their life, both at work and in personal settings. For instance, introverts may schedule periods during the workday for reduced verbal interactions, opting for email or text-based communication. When feasible, working from home can provide respite from bustling office environments. During commutes on public transportation, noise-canceling headphones can help create a quieter space. In shared living arrangements, retreating to a private bedroom with the door closed can offer solitude. These methods of isolation are valuable for introverts to recharge and prevent burnout. Still, it's essential to recognize that even introverts can benefit from some level of social support, albeit in smaller doses, to maintain a balanced life.

Extroverts may not be as affected by stress as introverts in the first place simply because of their personality. This is mainly due to their perception of stress and ability to function in a stimulating environment without feeling overstimulated. Also, their coping incorporates more social contact, which can positively influence emotional well-being. That said, engaging in extroverted behavior can be "mentally depleting" after three consecutive hours, according to a 2016 study.[4]

Extroverts may have so much enthusiasm for getting the job done that they become workaholics and burn out in the process. Extroverts may also be less likely to pick up on signs of stress or find it hard to talk to others about their emotional state, which can bring on burnout. In consideration of all these factors, extroverts can benefit from incorporating self-care, grounding, and relaxation for a more balanced approach and pay more attention to their emotions.

PROTECTING YOUR ENERGY

Once you've taken the time to incorporate self-care and focus on ways to energize your body, you'll need to be mindful of how to protect that energy. To do so successfully requires being conscious of how you feel energetically. Based on your energy level rather than on how many more items are on your to-do list, decide when you need to stop for the day. Those items will still be there tomorrow. And when others are asking you to do something, if you're tapped out, learn to say, "not today." Maybe you'll take it on tomorrow or next week. Perhaps you will say "no" altogether.

Another effective method for preserving your energy is by practicing self-compassion. Setting overly ambitious and unrealistic expectations for yourself can lead to inevitable disappointment, particularly if you place a high value on productivity. It can be tempting to perceive your shortcomings and failures as a reflection of your inadequacy.

It's important to recognize that self-criticism is not a constructive approach. It neither enhances your energy levels nor boosts your productivity. Instead, consider that the issue lies not in your inherent deficiencies but rather in having unrealistic expectations. Take a moment to recalibrate your expectations, embrace yourself at your current stage, and, if you have significant aspirations, grant yourself the time needed to achieve them

TABLE 26.1 Maintaining, Recovering, and Protecting Your Energy

Maintaining your energy
- Schedule time in your calendar for self-care.
- Create a red-velvet rope policy around your time.
- Avoid overscheduling yourself.

Recovering your energy
- Gauge your energy level.
- Avoid quick fixes.
- Create healthy habits (sleep, physical activity, nutrition, water intake, media consumption, nature, journaling, breathing, social support).

If you are an introvert:

- find activities that you can do alone or with one other person (e.g., taking a long walk, journaling, exercising).
- limit verbal contact and use email and text to communicate.
- work from home.
- use noise-canceling headphones on your commute and in a noisy office setting.
- get social support in small doses.

If you are an extrovert:

- surround yourself with others.
- focus on grounding and relaxation.
- notice what triggers you.
- pay attention to your emotions.

Protecting your energy
- Be aware of your energy levels.
- Take breaks as needed rather than focusing on your to-do list.
- Practice self-compassion.
- Readjust expectations to be realistic.

at a comfortable pace. Slow and steady progress can be the key to success.

CONCLUSION

Sustaining optimal energy levels is essential for overall well-being and productivity. This requires a combination of daily practices, mindful decision-making about future commitments, and effective recovery strategies for energy dips. To maintain your energy, establish consistent habits that support your health and prioritize self-care. Protecting your energy involves developing self-awareness, taking regular breaks, practicing self-compassion, and setting realistic expectations. By integrating these approaches, you can achieve a sustainable energy balance, enhance your well-being, and navigate the demands of daily life with greater ease, resilience, and vitality.

CHAPTER 27

Establishing Healthy Boundaries

Setting boundaries is an act of self-love.
OPRAH WINFREY, *THE WISDOM OF SUNDAYS*

While it's helpful to recover your energy when you are exhausted, you must take a preventative approach to protect it. One way to do this is to set appropriate boundaries.

We've established the importance of self-care and uncovered some of the main obstacles to implementing it, including poor time management, believing you don't deserve it, and overwhelming job demands. In fact, despite everything going on in the external world, self-care and overall boundary setting are not optional. Setting boundaries is the primary way to maintain your energy and well-being so you can be effective in your work and relationships.

In this section, we uncover the underlying beliefs, fears, and behaviors that lead to poor boundaries as well as 10 strategies for creating healthy ones.

LACK OF BOUNDARIES

If you are a giver, it won't surprise anyone much to find you in a helping profession. Perhaps you're a doctor, nurse, teacher, or therapist. You work hard all day providing care for others. You might stay at work until late, skip meals due to the high demands of your job, and even take your work home.

Maybe your career choice is less indicative of your giving tendency, and the way you relate to others in your life is more telling. Are you someone who gives away your time? When someone asks you for help, do you feel compelled to say "yes"?

The issues surrounding a lack of boundaries include control, fear, and low self-awareness. When you are so agreeable that you take on tasks you don't really want, you are letting other people control you. The reason behind this might be that you fear they will become angry or disappointed otherwise, and you care very much about how others feel. You may even consider it your job to make others happy. You might have a fear of rejection and try to please others so they stay close to you.

If you believe that your needs matter less than those of others, you will feel guilty about tending to your own needs and therefore prioritize other people's needs ahead of your own. The clearer you are about what you value and what you need, the more authentic you can be in your relationships and decision-making, and the more balanced you will be in your life.

When it comes to setting healthy boundaries, knowing yourself is key. Once you have clarity about what's important to you and what makes you tick, you can better manage your life and relate to others in a meaningful way.

THE PRICE OF OVER-GIVING

It's 4:35 p.m. on a Friday. Joanie approaches your desk. She asks if you could take a look at her report. She is nervous about meeting with the boss and hopes you can go over it with her and give her some pointers. You still have a lot of work to do yourself and you're looking forward to the weekend. You've worked hard all week. But how can you say "no"?

As you reflect on these instances of giving, you start to wonder when things might have taken a less favorable turn and why this happens.

Giving is a beautiful act. It allows you to contribute to the world and create connections with other people. Over-giving, on the other hand, is a sign of poor boundaries. We've already mentioned why you might be an over-giver, but what are the implications of this behavior?

Over time, you start to notice a shift. You feel depleted. You might even feel resentful when the sentiment isn't reciprocated. But there is a glue that keeps you coming back to give more.

The increase in positive feelings and the decrease in guilt are the two mechanisms that contribute to the perpetual cycle of over-giving. But this cycle is not sustainable (figure 27.1).

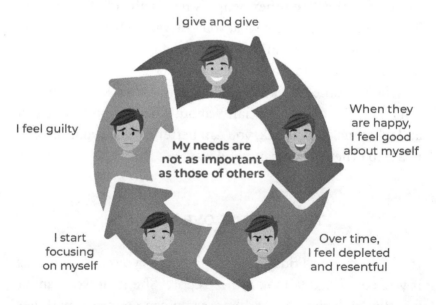

FIGURE 27.1 The nature of over-giving.

The story that exemplifies this scenario is *The Giving Tree* by Shel Silverstein. In it, a little boy and a tree have a beautiful relationship. The tree loves the boy and wants to fill his every desire. As the boy matures and grows into a man, his needs change and increase. The tree doesn't want to let the boy down. It continues to provide him with everything that he has. And as the book states, "The tree is happy." But eventually, the tree is left as a stump, having given away all its fruit, branches, and trunk to the boy. The story ends when the tree has nothing left to give and is "happy . . . but not really."[1]

You don't want to end up a tree stump no matter how much you care about others. At that point there won't be anything left to give, even if you want to. To break the cycle, you need to change your underlying belief about your worth. Recognize that over-giving is a source of self-neglect that can deplete your resources. Each time you need to decide about doing something for someone else, ask yourself, "What are the potential consequences of diverting my time and energy away from me?"

Set boundaries around your giving. Only once your own cup is overflowing can you give the excess away. Don't operate from an empty vessel. It only leads to burnout.

Create a boundary around your energy. Learn how at www .BurnoutToResilience.com.

DEBUNKING THE MYTHS ABOUT BOUNDARIES

There is a reason why you may not have good boundaries in place. It is essential that you examine your underlying beliefs and feelings. Here are some common myths about boundary setting and what keeps people from putting boundaries into place.

If I Decline Other People's Requests, They Will Be Angry with Me

While it may be true that some people will be angry with you some of the time, if you are dealing with reasonable people they will likely understand that you cannot always comply with their requests. Remember, people ask because they have nothing to lose, but just because they ask does not mean you have to say "yes." And, if someone is angry with you for setting a boundary, they are not respecting your needs. This is not the type of relationship you want to cultivate anyway.

People Won't Like Me If I Don't Do What They Want

The hope is that people will like you for who you are as a person, not for the favors you do for them. Be careful whom you attract into your life. Doing for others may be a way of pleasing them, but they won't necessarily like you for it. This conditions them to keep coming back and asking you for more favors because they know they can rely on you. While this is admirable, it does not necessarily lead to a reciprocal relationship. When you have unmet needs, you build up resentment.

Confrontation Is Scary—It's Easier to Say "Yes"

If you are scared by the idea of confrontation, this is part of your self-awareness. It's a first step to recognizing an area of weakness you need to work on continually. By improving your ability to stand up for your rights and negotiate what you want you will overcome the fear and establish motivation to forge ahead. The rewards will speak for themselves.

Sacrificing Myself for Others Makes Me a Good Person

Your deeds define part of who you are, and it's important to be generous and helpful. However, there needs to be a healthy limit to how much you give and how much you take for yourself. Self-sacrifice does not equate to being a better person. Instead, it is what leads to burnout over time.

If I Put Myself First, People Will Think I'm Selfish and Uncaring

When you ask for a favor, do you always expect the other person to say "yes"? If they don't, do you consider them selfish? It's time to reassess expectations of yourself and others. Perhaps you are a very empathic person, and when others struggle, you want to take care of them so much so that you lose track of your own needs. This is very selfless of you, but the opposite doesn't necessarily make you selfish. Remember, being focused on yourself is part of self-care. Without self-care, you are less capable of helping others in the long run.

Consider this definition of boundaries by psychologist David Gruder: "[A boundary] is any limit you need to honor to collaborate with another person without resentment and with integrity."[2] With these parameters as guidelines, you can make good decisions about when to say "yes."

HOW BOUNDARIES DECREASE DRAMA

When we don't have good boundaries in place, we fall into what Stephen Karpman calls the "Drama Triangle" (figure 27.2).[3] We take on one of three roles: the Victim, the Persecutor, or the Rescuer.

The role of the Victim is not for someone who receives poor treatment but someone who acts as if they are a victim. In this role, you recognize how desperately needy you are for not having met your needs for too long. You become passive and wait

FIGURE 27.2 The Drama Triangle. *Source*: Stephen B. Karpman, "Fairy Tales and Script Drama Analysis," *Transactional Analysis Bulletin* 7, no. 26 (1968): 39–43.

for someone else to step up to the plate and take care of you. When no one does, you either become angry and transition into a Persecutor or attempt being a Rescuer to someone else with the hope that the other person will eventually reciprocate.

As a Persecutor, you are finally releasing all your pent-up anger. The reason this role creates drama is that this person blames others for their problems rather than taking responsibility for himself. Following this release you are likely to experience guilt, which is an indication that your belief about your importance hasn't changed. The guilt then moves you back into the Rescuer role, where you get to compensate for lashing out.

The Rescuer believes their role is to rescue others. You put other people ahead of yourself, tend to focus on giving, and, consequently, don't ask for what you want or turn down other people's requests. The imbalance with which you approach others creates codependency because you approach relationships with a lose-win attitude. To have one of your needs met, you believe you need to give up something else. But no one can last forever in this depleting role. Over time, you build up resentment and may lash out as you transition into the role of the Persecutor. When abandoned, you may turn into a Victim.

This cycle continues, endlessly driven by feelings of anger, fear, and guilt. It never gets resolved, and the person continues to suppress their needs and suffer because of it. The only way out is to set boundaries.

If you think your life could benefit from putting boundaries into effect, here are 10 suggestions on how to set healthy boundaries with yourself and others:

1. Put a time limit on your work, whether at the office or home. Working late into the day does not allow you to recover from stress and can negatively affect your sleep. Give yourself a time cushion before bed to relax and unwind. This practice will help you feel more energized the next morning so you can give the work your all.

2. Decide when to stop receiving phone calls or checking emails. It's so easy for us to get carried away and think each notification from our phone is an urgent matter that needs immediate attention. Remember that although someone might reach out to you at all times of the day and night, you don't have to respond right away. When you need to focus on your tasks, turn off all notifications. When it's time to relax, turn off your devices.

3. Does your job expect you to work until the work is done? If so, consider how frequently you are willing to sacrifice your day off and for how long. When you decide ahead of time, you can set expectations with others and relieve yourself of the idea that you have to keep working regardless of your resources. The demands on you rarely ever end, but your weekends do.

4. You might be worried about letting your customers down if you don't respond to their every wish. Focus on reading their demands as requests. As in any relationship, it is feasible for you to be able to fulfill some requests and not others. Set realistic expectations with yourself and others on what you can and are willing to do.

5. If you are dealing with difficult personalities in your work or personal life, ask yourself how you want others to treat you. Sometimes our fear of losing out on a relationship pushes our boundary off the map. This only confirms to others that we have no limit in place and that they can get away with manipulating us to do what they want. Don't let your fear outweigh your values. Stay true to yourself. This will allow you to attract the right people rather than desperately attach yourself to the wrong ones.

6. When you're interacting with others, aim for respectful communication. Keep calm and excuse yourself if you need space rather than let your anger build. Similarly, don't engage with others who disrespect you. By setting clear expectations, you send a firm message that you will not tolerate yelling, blaming, or shaming.

7. Be clear on your values. This will allow you to make decisions more easily, especially when considering which tasks to take on. When someone makes a request of you, this sense of purpose that stems from your values can guide your decision on whether you accept or decline the request.

8. Before you take on a new task, let the other person know how much time you have. This sets a clear expectation of how long you can dedicate to the project and when you will stop. If it isn't a sufficient amount of time, this upfront clarity conversation can prevent you from taking on something you cannot realistically complete.

9. Assert yourself to protect your resources. If your boss or partner is asking you to take on a new project, share with them what you have on your plate already and prioritize together what this new project will replace. This ensures you don't overload yourself while providing support for new priorities that pop up.

10. Express your feelings appropriately. If someone else oversteps your boundary, you are likely to feel angry. Learn to express that anger in a way that describes the facts, connects their behavior to your feelings, and requests a change in approach from the other person. You will meet your needs more effectively in this way.

CONCLUSION

Setting boundaries may not be in your practice yet, but it is something you can put into effect with time. To be successful with boundary setting, you have to believe that you matter. Recognize that you have needs much like anyone else and that it is your responsibility to get your needs met. Also, realize that you have limited resources and that you need to protect those resources from depletion by being strategic about how much of them you give away and how much you keep for yourself.

When you believe you matter, you can sidestep guilt. You can tune into your values and make purpose-driven decisions about what you do with your time and how you interact with other people. You feel empowered to ask for what you do want and to say "no" to what you don't.

We place white picket fences around our homes to protect our property. It's time we recognize the need to do the same with our resources so we can have more balance between our internal needs and the external demands placed on us.

CHAPTER 28

Transitioning Out of Work Mode

When we talk about energy, self-care, and setting healthy boundaries, we need to focus not only on what happens at the office but what happens in our personal lives. As you transition out of work, you need to consider what practices will help you do so most effectively so you can maximize your recovery time.

CREATING A TRANSITION FROM WORK TO PERSONAL LIFE IN THE REMOTE WORK ERA

In the post-pandemic world, the line between work and personal life has become increasingly blurred for many. With remote work becoming the norm, the physical act of leaving the office no longer serves as a clear boundary. This new reality presents unique challenges in separating professional responsibilities from personal time, especially for those juggling family life alongside work duties.

To maintain a healthy work-life balance in this new context, it's crucial to create intentional transitions that allow you to mentally "clock out" and fully engage in your personal life. Without these boundaries, work stress can easily seep into your home life, potentially affecting relationships, health, and emotional well-being.

Here are five strategies to help you create a transition out of work mode, even when your office is just steps away from your living space:

1. *Create a "virtual commute"*: Set aside time at the end of your workday for a short walk outside or around your home. This mimics the act of leaving a physical office and helps signal to your brain that work is over.

2. *Establish an end-of-work ritual*: Develop a routine that marks the end of your workday. This could involve shutting down your work computer, closing the door to your home office (if you have one), or changing out of your "work clothes" into more comfortable attire.

3. *Practice mindfulness*: Take a few minutes to ground yourself through deep breathing exercises or a short meditation session. This can help clear your mind of work-related thoughts and prepare you for personal time.

4. *Use technology to your advantage*: Set up automatic "out of office" responses or status updates on your work communication tools at the end of your designated work hours. This helps reinforce boundaries with colleagues and clients.

5. *Create a relaxing environment*: Transform your space from "work mode" to "home mode" by adjusting lighting, playing soothing music, or using aromatherapy. These sensory cues can help shift your mindset away from work.

Additional considerations for remote workers:

- Designate a specific work area. If possible, have a dedicated workspace that you can physically leave at the end of the day.
- Set and communicate clear working hours. Let your team know when you're available and when you're off the clock.
- Use separate devices or accounts for work and personal use to minimize the temptation to check work emails during personal time.
- Schedule regular breaks throughout the day to prevent burnout and maintain productivity.

Remember, in a remote work environment, the responsibility for creating work-life boundaries often falls more heavily on the individual. By implementing these strategies and being mindful of the need for clear transitions, you can protect your personal time and energy, leading to better overall well-being and job satisfaction.

As with any significant change, adapting to this new way of working may take time. Be patient with yourself and adjust these strategies as needed to find what works best for your unique situation. Additionally, consider discussing with your employer any support or resources they can provide to help maintain a healthy work-life balance in this new normal.

HOW TO TAKE VACATIONS FROM A BUSY JOB

Even if you're aware of the benefits of taking a vacation from work, there may be real obstacles that make it challenging to

---

TABLE 28.1 Transitioning from Work to Home

Physical Recharge:

- *Engage in a brief physical activity*: Even a short walk, stretch, or yoga pose can help reduce physical tension and mental fatigue.
- *Practice relaxation techniques*: Deep breathing, meditation, or progressive muscle relaxation can help calm the mind and body.

Mental Shift:

- *Change your environment*: Physically separate yourself from your workspace.
- *Change your attire*: Put on comfortable clothing to signal the end of the workday.
- *Mindful transition*: Spend a few minutes focusing on your breath and present moment awareness.

Emotional Processing:

- *Journaling*: Briefly jot down any work-related thoughts or concerns to clear your mind.
- *Talk it out*: Share your thoughts and feelings with a friend, family member, or therapist.

---

step away. According to the U.S. Travel Association's 2018 study, American workers used an average of 17.4 vacation days that year. However, this falls short of the historical average of 20.3 days used annually between 1976 and 2000.[1]

The study identified two distinct groups of workers: "homebodies," who use few vacation days for travel, and "megatravelers," who use most of their time off for trips. Interestingly, mega-travelers reported significantly higher levels of happiness compared to homebodies (see figure 28.1). This find-

- Greater happiness
- Greater work satisfaction
- Increased likelihood of a promotion
- Greater recovery from stress
- Increased physical health
- Have more fun
- Create more lasting memories

- Appear more dedicated
- Stay on top of workload
- Play it safe
- Save money
- Maintain routine

FIGURE 28.1   Project time off. *Source*: U.S. Travel Association, 2018.

ing demonstrates that using vacation time for travel can have a substantial positive impact on overall well-being.

While more recent data on these specific groups isn't available, a 2022 report shows that the trend of underutilizing vacation time has continued. More than half of Americans (55 percent) didn't use all of their paid time off in 2022, a 27.8 percent increase from 2018. This suggests that the challenges of taking time off persist, possibly exacerbated by the rise of remote work and the blurring of work-life boundaries.

It's important to note that not all workers follow a typical Monday-to-Friday schedule. For those with alternative work schedules, planning vacations can be more complex. Federal guidelines for "in lieu of" holidays provide some insight into how nonstandard schedules are accommodated. For instance, employees on alternative work schedules (AWS) are entitled to "in lieu of" holidays when a holiday falls on their regular day off.[2]

CONQUER BURNOUT AND RECHARGE WITH STRATEGIC VACATIONS

Planning vacations in advance is your weapon against burnout and a gateway to the joys of time off. This proactive approach isn't just about happiness with loved ones; it gives you something to eagerly anticipate. Scheduling your break creates a mental separation between work and personal life.

Clear communication is your key to a smooth vacation exit. Let colleagues know your absence dates and who will handle your responsibilities. This transparency keeps workflows flowing and eases worries about your workload during your absence.

Don't forget your clients! Inform them of your upcoming vacation and provide alternative contacts for assistance. Many clients appreciate your time off, especially if they value long-term relationships over immediate availability.

Preparation is king when it comes to minimizing vacation disruptions. Tie up loose ends before you leave to ensure a smooth transition for yourself and your team. This might involve completing projects or delegating tasks that require attention while you're away.

Finally, for a truly rejuvenating vacation, disconnect digitally. Turn off work notifications on your devices to resist the urge to check in. This is especially important in a remote work environment where boundaries can easily blur.

For those with nonstandard work schedules, a little extra planning might be needed. Coordinate with your employer about how holidays and vacation times are handled for your specific schedule. Be flexible and choose quieter periods in your work cycle for vacations.

The U.S. Travel Association study found a surprising link: those who travel more are not only happier with their company and job but are also more likely to receive promotions. This challenges the myth that constant availability is the key to career advancement.

By taking proactive steps to use your vacation days and truly disconnect from work, regardless of your schedule, you can recharge, gain fresh perspectives, and ultimately become a more effective contributor in the long run. Don't let the fear of work piling up or seeming less dedicated prevent you from enjoying the numerous benefits of a well-deserved break. This approach, presented in clear steps, empowers you to successfully take vacations from even the busiest job.

HOW TO MAKE YOUR NEXT VACATION COUNT IN THE POST-PANDEMIC ERA

In today's world of remote work and flexible schedules, the concept of "vacation" has evolved. For many, the lines between work and personal time have blurred, making it even more crucial to intentionally disconnect and recharge. Whether you're a traditional 9-to-5 worker, a remote employee, or someone with a nontraditional schedule, vacationing can be both rejuvenating and potentially stressful. The key is to ensure that your vacation meets your specific needs and work situation.

Advanced planning remains essential, but flexibility is now more important than ever. Post-pandemic travel often involves additional considerations such as health and safety protocols, potential travel restrictions, and the need for contingency plans. Set realistic expectations and be prepared for last-minute changes. Pack not only weather-appropriate clothing but also any necessary work equipment if you're planning a "workcation." For remote workers, this might include noise-canceling headphones, portable chargers, or a mobile hotspot.

Choose your travel companions wisely, especially if you're planning an extended stay or workcation. For those with non-traditional schedules, coordinating time off with travel partners might require extra planning. Remember, being away from your routines can be stressful, particularly for remote workers who may already have a less structured daily life.

According to the U.S. Travel Association's "Paid Time Off Trends Fact Sheet," certain industries view travel as a way to reduce stress and avoid burnout. For example, individuals working in business services or health care industries were more motivated to travel to avoid burnout.[3] While this study doesn't specifically address remote workers, it's reasonable to extrapolate that traveling can be a stress-busting option for many professionals, including those working from home. In the post-pandemic world, where many have experienced increased work demands and decreased autonomy, taking time off for travel can provide a much-needed change of scenery and break from routine. This can be especially valuable for remote workers who may struggle with the blurred lines between work and home life.

However, be cautious of overscheduling your trip. The temptation to see everything can be strong, especially for remote workers who might feel they need to maximize their time away from their home office. Balance adventure with relaxation. For those with flexible schedules, consider spreading out your vacation days to create longer weekends rather than taking one extended break. This approach can help maintain work continuity while still providing regular opportunities to recharge.

Accommodation choices have become even more critical in the post-pandemic era. For remote workers or those on nontraditional schedules, having a comfortable workspace within your vacation rental can be crucial. Home-sharing options or extended-stay hotels often provide the space and amenities needed to balance work and leisure effectively. Look for accommodations with reliable Wi-Fi, dedicated workspaces, and quiet areas for video calls if you need to check in with work.

For families, especially those with parents working remotely or on shift schedules, having separate spaces for work, sleep, and play can make a significant difference in the quality of the vacation. Consider rentals with multiple rooms or hotel suites that allow for privacy and flexibility in daily routines.

Lastly, set clear boundaries between work and vacation time, even if you're on a workcation. Designate specific hours for work tasks and stick to them. Use the rest of your time to fully engage

---

TABLE 28.2   **Making the Most of Your Vacation**

- Set realistic expectations.
- Pack weather-appropriate, comfortable clothing.
- Travel with someone with whom you get along.
- Don't make too many plans for one day.
- Plan for days of adventure and days of relaxation.
- Stay in accommodations that afford you space.

in your surroundings and activities. For those with nontraditional schedules, communicate your availability clearly with both your work team and travel companions to manage expectations.

Thoughtfully plan your next vacation with these considerations in mind, and you will create a truly rejuvenating experience that caters to your unique work-life situation in the post-pandemic world.

CONCLUSION

The line between work and personal life has blurred in the post-pandemic era, especially for remote workers. To maintain a healthy work-life balance, create intentional transitions that allow you to mentally "clock out." Designate a specific workspace, set clear working hours, and use separate devices for work and personal use. Practice mindfulness techniques, engage in relaxing activities, and set clear boundaries with colleagues. Remember, taking vacations and truly disconnecting is crucial for long-term well-being. By implementing these strategies you can protect your personal time and energy, leading to better overall well-being and job satisfaction.

Exercise for Step 5

The goal of this two-part exercise is to increase your energy. The first part involves overcoming mindset obstacles; the second involves committing to implementing aspects of your self-care regimen.

Step 1: If you don't have self-care incorporated into your life, it is likely that you aren't making the time for it and that you don't believe you are worth it. On a scale of 0–100 (where 0 = not at all and 100 = absolutely true), how much do you believe you are worthy of self-care? _____

If you scored 69 or below, practice the affirmation "I am worth it" every day throughout the day and come back to re-rate your belief on the 100-point scale once weekly until you've reached a score of at least 70. Then move on to step 2. If you scored 70 or above, move on to step 2 now.

Step 2: Consider which self-care activities you would benefit from incorporating in your life now that you believe you deserve it. Start with the basics (e.g., getting a full night of sleep, eating healthy meals, exercising your body several days a week, taking breaks throughout the workday). When you're ready to upgrade, you can start to implement meditation, massages, hot baths, or other relaxing and fun activities as well as plan for future travel.

I commit to implementing these self-care strategies:

_____

_____

_____

_____

_____

_____

This is my plan for when and how I will incorporate these into my routine:

_____

_____

_____

_____

_____

_____

Effort

*Workaholics aren't heroes. They don't save the day,
they just use it up. The real hero is home because
they figured out a faster way.*

JASON FRIED AND DAVID HEINEMEIER HANSSON, *REWORK*

An attempt to do something, especially when it's difficult, is often equated with overexertion and burnout. But this definition misses a crucial point: effort doesn't always have to be hard. In this section, we'll explore two approaches to effort. The first is related to the concept of "work smarter, not harder," which indicates that there is a way to attain results without overexerting yourself. The second relates to the concept of *Right Effort*, which is part of the Buddhist Eightfold Path to enlightenment.

CHAPTER 29

Smart Effort

When you think about it, effort is something that requires motivation. You put your energy into tasks because you are either moving toward something you want or away from something you wish to avoid. So when we talk about effort, keep in mind the rewards that are swaying your decisions.

Once you have a clear understanding of the rewards you seek, you must know how to focus your efforts to be balanced. Weak attention means a lack of effort, which is likely to keep the status quo at best. Too intense an effort will drain you. Instead, the goal is to engage in your work and find joy in it. You may have to challenge your beliefs about what is possible for you to achieve without overexerting yourself.

WHAT MOTIVATES YOU TO DO A GOOD JOB?

Imagine a stranger comes up to you with an intriguing proposal: "I have a set of tasks for you to complete, and I'm willing to pay you for your time. I'd like you to dedicate at least one-third of your day to these tasks in exchange for compensation."

How would you react to such an offer? Naturally, you'd have a multitude of questions swirling in your mind: What specific tasks are you asking me to do? Is there a maximum daily time commitment beyond the minimum of eight hours? And, of course, how much compensation are we talking about here?

These questions examine whether there is a good effort-reward balance because your time is your most precious resource. You want to spend your time on optimally rewarding tasks. To help you understand what you find motivating, you need to examine the different types of rewards associated with work and identify which rewards are most essential based on your values.

Before we jump in, let's take a look at what motivation is and what is behind it.

WHAT IS MOTIVATION?

Each of your actions has a reason, or motive, for it. You have desires or needs that cause you to behave in a certain way. Whether you move toward a target or away from it will depend on your motives.

You are faced with choices each day, even if you don't recognize them. The reason you often overlook this fact is that you have fallen into a routine, but completing a set of tasks or doing nothing at all is still a choice. The question is, what leads you to continue doing something, and, similarly, what can get you to change?

Human beings are inherently creatures of habit. When we become accustomed to a certain way of doing things, it feels more effortless. The learning curve is flattened, and our attention requirements decrease. This phenomenon is often referred to as "maintaining the status quo." If you find contentment in your current situation because of the actions you've taken, you're likely to stick to your established routine. The motivation behind this inclination may arise from the satisfaction derived from your present circumstances, a fear of change, or a desire to conserve energy by minimizing effort.

It is when you want something more that you are required to change. If you want a raise at work, to expand your social circle, or to lose weight, you need to focus your efforts on what will get you the results associated with your goal.

And while attaining the goal is sometimes the reward for your efforts, there are several other ways you can feel rewarded for your work.

TYPES OF REWARDS

Motivation serves as the driving force behind your actions, guiding your behavior toward an anticipated outcome. It's this deliberate intention that propels you into action. For instance, if you find yourself unemployed and your goal is to earn money, your job search becomes a focused effort aimed at achieving your financial objective.

But once you land the job and you have a guaranteed paycheck, different motivations are needed to do the work. If you've experienced intense stress on the job or even burnout, you need to take a step back and think about what you're doing and why you're doing it.

Beyond the paycheck, you chose this line of work and continue to choose it each day by showing up. There must be more keeping you there. By getting clear on your motivations and how they align with your values, you can take inventory of whether you are in your power or need to redesign your work life.

There are two types of rewards that keep us motivated to work: external and internal.

External Rewards

Returning to our earlier example, what we often focus on initially is external because it is central to our survival. We seek work, especially early in our career, that will pay the bills. When we are more advanced in our careers, we may want a promotion in title and pay.

Other rewards that keep us motivated to do our work every day include feedback, acknowledgment, and recognition. As humans we have a need to feel seen. If we work hard on a project, we want to know that our efforts are noticed. When we receive praise or even some direction on how to improve, we feel like we are making an impact and that our hard work amounts to something.

In the movie *Hidden Figures*, Katherine G. Johnson works relentlessly at her NASA job. Her brilliant mind focuses on calculating orbital mechanics necessary to perform a successful spaceflight. No matter how hard or long she works, she is often unable to stay ahead of the curve. As soon as she hands in her documents, she is told that the team is moving in a different direction.[1]

If this were your reality, perhaps at first you would feel frustrated for having wasted your efforts. But if this were a pattern at your job, chances are that the pay would not be enough to keep you there because once you've met your basic needs, what drives you is internal.

Internal Rewards

What keeps Johnson working as hard as she does is the knowledge that she is part of something monumental. The meaning she derives from NASA's mission is so great that it allows her to keep forging ahead.

It takes a while for all of Johnson's efforts to amount to anything concrete, but when the first American astronauts complete their roundtrip flight to space, she feels an immense sense of pride.

Despite many roadblocks, Katherine Johnson's determination pays off in many internal and external rewards. But not all work obstacles are solved by effort alone. So how do we know when to stick it out and when to move on?

When the Rewards Aren't Motivating Enough

If you were making half a million dollars a year in your career in your early thirties and were a vice president already, would you quit your job? It may sound counterintuitive, but as demonstrated in the story of Greg Smith, external rewards are often not enough.

Greg Smith was vice president of the investment firm Goldman Sachs. After 12 years he decided to leave despite his title and high compensation. The three main reasons he cited for his departure included the company's declining "integrity," a "toxic" environment, and the company's culture of "ripping" off clients. While the external rewards were motivating, the lack of alignment between the company's values and his own took their toll.[2]

My cousin also worked for Goldman Sachs in the early 2000s. During one of my stays at his New York apartment, I watched him wake up very early and leave for work, not to return until 10:00 or 11:00 p.m. He described using his apartment only for sleeping and showering on weekdays because he would be working all day at the office and then dining out with clients each night.

While he was being compensated well for his time, the pressure to perform was even higher. The company had high expectations, and as happens when one is in sales, the ultimate decision to buy lies with the prospective customer. The stress was mounting, and I found my cousin resorting to pills to deal with his anxiety and slow mental deterioration. Eventually, he realized the external rewards were inadequate when compared to how the demands of the job affected him, and he quit.

Why Rewards Are Important

We've already mentioned that rewards motivate us to work, but there is more to it than that. My research has uncovered seven answers to the question, "Why are rewards important?"

1. *Boosting self-efficacy*: Rewards play a critical role in reinforcing our belief in our ability to perform tasks effectively. Christina Maslach, in her article "Burned-Out," highlights that the key factors influencing efficacy on the job are control and reward. In other words, having autonomy in your decisions and receiving recognition or compensation for your efforts both enhance your confidence in your capabilities and improve your performance.

2. *Engagement*: Research shows that employees who are highly engaged in their work experience significantly more rewards compared to their exhausted and less engaged colleagues.[4] This finding highlights the cyclical relationship between engagement and rewards. When we have the energy to perform well and enter a state of flow, we are more likely to perceive our work as meaningful. The rewards we receive as a result of this engagement reinforce our efforts, motivating us to maintain and deepen our involvement over time.

3. *Feeling valued*: Whether the reward is internal or external, when you work hard, you want to be compensated for your efforts. When you are acknowledged

verbally, financially, or otherwise, you feel like others respect and value your work. This motivates you to keep going.

4. *Intrinsic satisfaction*: While external rewards can certainly boost morale, it's the internal sense of accomplishment and purpose that truly drives long-term engagement. When we feel connected to our work, experience a sense of autonomy, and see the direct impact of our efforts, we are intrinsically motivated. This intrinsic reward system fuels our passion, creativity, and overall job satisfaction.

5. *Self-worth*: When you receive adequate rewards for your efforts, not only does the recognition justify the work but it elevates your sense of self. Success comes from putting your efforts toward a task and learning from your failures. Once you have an accomplishment you feel good about yourself, and this motivates you to keep learning and striving.

6. *Trust*: As you probably already know, trust is critical in any relationship. The relationship you have with your organization is no exception. For that to happen, you need to feel like it fulfills its promises. If the higher-ups in your organization recognize your work and reward you accordingly you build trust, which continues to motivate you to do good work for them.

7. *Inspiration*: One source of reward is positive feedback. When you put your energy toward accomplishing a company goal, getting feedback on your work can feel empowering. It helps build up your self-efficacy, and it inspires you to continue on your journey because someone is watching and supporting you.

Rewards are essential for a variety of reasons. Regardless of what those reasons are for you, the most important aspect to keep in mind is that the rewards you receive are adequate for the work you are doing. You may be making a half a million dollars as Smith did, but if there is a misalignment between your values and that of your company, the pay alone won't likely keep you there. That said, while rewards don't lessen the workload, they can help stave off burnout because of the motivation they instill in you.

With that in mind, let's consider what is needed for you to have effort-rewards balance.

BALANCED REWARDS

When we seek balance, we look for ways to engage without too much or too little effort and to have our efforts amount to meaningful rewards. We already know that too much effort can lead to burnout. Let's now take a look at what happens when there is too little reward.

Researchers asked students to do a mind-numbingly boring task: screwing bolts for an hour. Afterward, they offered some students $1 and others $20 to recommend the task to friends. Those who were paid $20 felt justified in lying. They reasoned that the high pay made the boring task worthwhile. So, without feeling any guilt, they recommended the task to others. The students who received only $1 experienced cognitive dissonance when asked to recommend the task to others. They felt a tension between their belief that the task was monotonous and their decision to support it. Because their compensation was too small to justify lying, they had to change their perception of the task to eliminate their inner conflict.[5]

If you are giving your job your all and aren't getting the rewards you desire, you might convince yourself that the job must be worth it. Alternatively, you might take matters into your own hands to seek fairness.

In the study "Interplay between Job Demands and Job Resources," researchers found that employees whose job required high effort but provided low reward called in sick more often than any other employees.[6] We can interpret their absence as a result of being sick, as a lack of motivation to come to work, or as a way to reward themselves for their high effort by taking time off. Sickness may relate to burnout, especially if the sickness is psychosomatic or a result of job-related stress. Taking time off, by contrast, might be an attempt to balance the relationship between effort and reward.

Rather than having to explain away your reasons for staying in a dead-end situation or sabotaging your career, consider some ways to balance the equation.

Increase rewards. Approach your employer for higher rewards. Remember that rewards come in a variety of forms, so while you may not always be able to get increased monetary compensation, you can probably attain additional sources of reward (e.g., a promotion in title, more vacation days, a work-from-home day, stock in the company).

Recognize if you are not being compensated fairly and address this with your hiring manager. If they are unwilling or unable to rectify the situation, take proactive action and start your job search. It's a good idea to know what the market will bear and get what you are worth.

Decrease demands. Employers are in the business of making money, and their biggest cost is employee salaries. It is natural for them to try to get as much as possible from their hires, but they need to recognize there is a limit to how much they can get away with. Aim to turn down anything that doesn't align with your long-term career goals so you can produce quality work on fewer items rather than have your hand in an overwhelming number of tasks that are half-baked.

Become empowered. In *The Truth about Burnout*, Christina Maslach and Michael Leiter recommend systematizing your autonomy, finding ways to keep yourself accountable, and creating relative rewards for your work.[7] Let's break this down.

- Systematizing your autonomy means establishing structured processes or routines that allow you to have more control over your work while maintaining accountability. This creates a framework that enables you to take ownership of your tasks and responsibilities without feeling overwhelmed.

- Keeping yourself accountable involves setting clear goals, tracking your progress, and regularly assessing your performance. This ensures you stay on track and meet your objectives, thus reducing the risk of burnout.

- Creating relative rewards for your work means recognizing your achievements and rewarding yourself in a way that is meaningful to you. Doing so can boost your motivation and job satisfaction.

These steps give you the ability to address issues as they come up. If your manager tends to micromanage, talk about how this negatively affects you and what would better allow you to do your work.

Balancing rewards is not only relevant when you feel under-motivated. It is also applicable when you are over-motivated or motivated by fear.

Set clear boundaries. One of my coaching clients made it her mission to rebalance the effort-reward equation. Catalina, a physician and researcher, had a tendency of taking on too much for fear of missing out or of being perceived in a negative light. She came to see me because she felt overwhelmed with work demands and resented her predicament.

As a result of our work, she was able to establish helpful criteria of when to say "no" to others' requests and reward herself in the process. For each request she turned down, she paid herself $100—money she could use on a shopping spree. Very quickly, the motivation to say "no" outweighed the motivation to say "yes," and Catalina not only had less stress but also more downtime.

She also established a checklist of when to say "yes" to requests. This list reflected her values and priorities. If the effort was low (e.g., someone requested her to give a talk she'd already given and therefore didn't need to spend a lot of time preparing for it), she would be more likely to take it on, but only if she got paid and didn't already have more than three other travel commitments for the year.

By establishing clear guidelines for how to handle incoming requests, you too can avoid feeling overwhelmed, guilty, or resentful. Be clear on your values and the available time before you commit yourself to anything extra.

Focus on meaning. Rather than trying to get more rewards by taking on excessive amounts of work, focus your efforts and find value by going more in depth with the projects you already have. By becoming engaged, your job starts to feel more meaningful. If the work you are doing is not challenging enough, communicate your needs to your supervisor. By focusing on meaningless work, you lose out on an opportunity to increase your professional development.

Recover your energy. If you are burned out, you may be attempting to conserve your energy by neglecting responsibilities. Focus on recovering your energy and then figure out whether you can reengage with your work in a different, more effective way that maintains your vitality.

Knowing how much effort you put in versus the reward you get can help you maintain a balanced life. If you feel unbalanced, use this knowledge to make adjustments. Remember, you have the power to create a balanced life.

Once you've secured adequate rewards and have garnered the motivation to work, it's time to consider the effort side of the equation.

BALANCED EFFORT

It takes effort to make things happen, and putting too little or too much effort into your work can take you out of balance.

Previously we said that too little effort could be a way of compensating yourself when you feel undercompensated. You might also find that with too little effort you are underperforming. You need to understand why you engage in your work in the way you do and figure out how to become better aligned with your inner rewards.

When your attention is weak, your performance will suffer. What leads to poor attention is external distractions, inner attachments, fears, and desires. To improve your attention so your efforts amount to the desired outcome, it's important to eliminate distractions.

External chaos (emails, alerts on your phone, or a messy desk) can break up your concentration and prevent you from focusing your efforts. Take the necessary steps to minimize notifications, set expectations about your availability, and clear out any clutter.

Even with a perfectly controlled environment, chaos can ensue internally. You might be overthinking your decisions, be filled with doubt and skepticism, or feel afraid of what the future might hold. If you find it difficult to pay attention, it might be because there is something you are avoiding. Practice controlling your mind through meditation to bring your best self to work. Focus on gratitude for everything that's right in your life now rather than worrying about what's to come. This will keep you in the present and improve your attention at work.

The problem may not lie in your attention, but in your beliefs about how much effort you need to exert. You may feel exhausted by all the responsibilities you are already carrying and overwhelmed by the prospect of taking on anything else. But consider this: Life doesn't have to be difficult.

Your beliefs are what drive your behaviors, and if you believe your work has to be difficult, you may either find yourself struggling or resisting it altogether. By using the power of the mind, you can focus on attaining what you want and perhaps making it easier than you would otherwise estimate it to be.

If you've ever experienced a state of flow, you know that you can exert a lot of effort and not feel drained. Optimal engagement enables you to gain confidence, feel grateful, and come into harmony with your efforts.

Tools such as visualization can be helpful for achieving goals more smoothly. Once you see yourself having the success that you want, going through the motions in real life is less daunting. Moreover, there have been countless reports from people who have used their spirituality to achieve goals in less time and with less effort. The law of attraction states that when you

TABLE 29.1 **Creating Effort-Reward Balance**

Consider which part of the effort-reward equation lacks balance and use the table below as a guide for increasing balance on either side.

To Balance Rewards	To Balance Efforts
Increase Rewards • Celebrate accomplishments, no matter how small. • Seek positive feedback and appreciation.	*Reduce Demands* • Prioritize tasks and delegate when possible. • Learn to say no to additional responsibilities.
Empower Yourself • Set clear goals and break them down into smaller steps. • Develop your skills and knowledge.	*Streamline Processes* • Eliminate unnecessary tasks and distractions. • Create a productive work environment.
Recover Energy • Practice mindfulness and relaxation techniques. • Prioritize sleep and healthy habits.	*Cultivate a Positive Mindset* • Challenge negative thoughts and beliefs. • Practice gratitude and focus on the positive.

focus on what you want rather than on what you don't want, you can attract the right things to you.[8]

CONCLUSION

Smart effort is all about a balanced relationship between effort and rewards. Rewards are what motivate you to work and are important because they drive you to do your job. The more engaged you are, the more likely you will accomplish great results, which increase your efficacy and encourage you to keep striving. Rewards, when adequate in relation to your efforts, make you feel valued. Without them you can quickly burn out.

While hard work and dedication are essential, they are not the only factors contributing to success. To maximize your efforts, focus on increasing your efficiency and productivity. By creating a focused work environment and engaging deeply in your tasks, you can achieve more in less time. Additionally, by aligning your thoughts and intentions with your goals, you can harness the power of the law of attraction to manifest your desired outcomes. When you combine focused action with mindful intention, you can accelerate your progress and achieve greater success.

CHAPTER 30

Right Effort

In Buddhism, eight guidelines can lead to enlightenment. They are known collectively as the Eightfold Path.[1] While our focus here is more on getting through the workday with balance rather than on reaching enlightenment, there is wisdom in the way Buddhists conceptualize effort.

Right effort is one of the concepts in the Eightfold Path. What is meant by right effort is mental discipline: the ability to prevent and release negative thoughts and feelings and, instead, cultivate and strengthen good thoughts and qualities. By being aware of your inner experience, you can establish habits that transform, empower, and strengthen you.

Any growth takes time and effort, whether it's personal, professional, or spiritual. If you are impatient with the process, you will become frustrated. Recognize that while you think you want the transformation to happen quickly, you may not be able to handle it all at once. When it unfolds slowly over time, you have an opportunity to adapt. The ultimate reward that comes from this transformation and growth is freedom.

RELATIVE MOTIVE STRENGTH

There exists a continuum that spans between achievement motivation (AM), characterized by the drive toward reaching your desired goal, and failure avoidance or fear of failure (FF), marked

FIGURE 30.1 Relative Motive Strength.

by a tendency to retreat from your desired goal due to fear. This continuum is referred to as Relative Motive Strength (RMS; figure 30.1). When you position yourself closer to the achievement end of this spectrum, you tend to connect your efforts on challenging tasks with positive outcomes using terms such as "dedication," "concentration," "commitment," and "success." Conversely, when you lean more toward FF, your efforts on demanding tasks are more likely to be associated with negative outcomes, including feelings of being "overloaded," "stressed," and "obsessed," as well as experiencing burnout.[2]

When you think about what is behind the difference between these two extremes, it's the way you see yourself. Self-efficacy is the belief that you can be successful. Your self-efficacy can be affected by your overarching core belief about personal adequacy or can be task-specific. Either way, it's an illustration that when faced with demands from the external world, your thinking can shape how you perceive those demands and yourself.

When you see yourself as adequate, you don't allow your failures to define you. You understand the importance of your long-term goals and that failure is part of the learning process. This keeps you motivated and unafraid. Alternatively, when you fear failure to the point of short-changing your efforts, you see yourself as inadequate and want to avoid this pain point, which will confirm your beliefs. In short, it's about your inner dialogue, your self-judgment.

Both the AM and the FF individuals have a goal. The former is more focused on achievement. The latter is more focused on avoiding failure. Their actions will be different because of their varying focal points, and their success rates will, therefore, vary as well. It's easy to see why FF individuals enter into a self-fulfilling prophecy when their lack of success becomes attributed to their inadequacies. This wrongful attribution reinforces their avoidance of demanding tasks, thus linking their past, present, and future (figure 30.2).

Most individuals fall somewhere in the middle of the RMS continuum. And if you are a perfectionist, you can end up on either end. That means that you may be able to reach great heights, but it will be at a cost—namely, to your state of balance.

So how can you achieve greatness and still be balanced? How can you attain success without burning out in the process? One answer to this dilemma lies in ancient philosophy.

FIGURE 30.2 Self-fulfilling prophecy.

PASSIVE PRESENCE: THE ART OF NON-DOING

Over 2,500 years ago, in present-day Nepal, a monk began teaching what came to be known as the Middle Way. This monk, now known as Buddha, taught that the Middle Way was how one could be free from living in extremes.[3] His teachings challenge much of how Westerners run their businesses and their lives.

Many of us, including high aimers and perfectionists, focus on what we can do. We busy our days with lists of tasks to accomplish and seem never to have enough time to get everything done. Living in this way is very stressful. We can feel buried by our work, so we start to multitask with the hope that we will get more done. Working on multiple tasks at once only makes us fall out of balance, and because it entails distraction, we can become confused about what's most important. It's better to do less at once, attain mastery, and then move on.

According to Buddhism, doing is the way of limitation. It's filled with our thoughts and judgments and creates a world of pleasure and pain. Instead, Buddhism proposes *action without doing*. We have to get beyond our thoughts, and that will make our actions perfect.

There are two targets in this art of non-doing. First, we look at what not to do. This helps us eliminate tasks from our list rather than continually add more. It helps us focus on what's most important rather than multitask and lose our integrity. This also includes not thinking and judging, which prevent us from acting. This philosophy is in line with the saying that "less is more."

Second, we focus on how to do without doing. So, rather than swimming against the current, allow the current to lead you. Every sailor knows that using the power of the wind can move the boat more forcefully in the direction they want rather than opposing the wind's strength. This translates into being flexible in your thinking and actions and building momentum on the existing structures around you.

Recall the first time you learned how to drive. There were so many aspects to think about. You may have wondered, "How do people make it look so easy?" You had to be very focused to avoid making mistakes, to make sure you were safe, and to follow all the rules. It may have felt overwhelming to simultaneously think about signaling while changing lanes, about slowing down with adequate space to not hit the driver at the stop sign in front of you, or about merging onto the highway when there were fast-moving cars flying by. But with lots of practice, your mental focus lessened. Now that you've mastered driving, you likely have days that you get to work and don't even remember how you got there.

There are two lessons in this example. The first is that mastery comes with time and consistent practice, but until then, you need a lot of mental energy. You may need to focus on a strategy to get things done. With mastery, you can get into the flow and engage in the task without being overly focused on it. You become one with the action.

The second lesson is that when you fall into habits, you can end up engaging in tasks mindlessly. However, this is quite different from non-doing. The main difference is awareness. Non-doing is doing with consciousness, which is different from unconscious action. It is intentional and comes from letting go of your thoughts and feelings, which cloud your awareness.

According to the spiritual teacher Samvara, you can achieve perfection through a formula:

Tremendous Attention + Extreme Abandonment
= Perfect Action.[4]

He refers to being very mindful and focused rather than having mere thoughts. It is about taking action without focusing on the outcome. It's like aiming your arrow at a target, pulling back the bow, and then letting the arrow go. You can't hit the goal unless you release the arrow. Similarly, you have to be hyper-focused on what you want, take action, and then let go so you can move on to the next perfect action without judgment, worry, or fear about the outcome of the previous action.

It's about turning off the struggle. When you're faced with a problem, head into the solution, rather than looking for excuses or for someone to blame. Problem-solving in this way differs substantially from obsessing over details, ruminating, and becoming paralyzed and from staying stuck in your mind. This is a way of doing but having little to show for it. As Samvara said in his lecture "How to Do Buddhism," "When you're doing, the shadow of the self is cast over everything."[5] By this, he is referring to the ego. This is when we get caught up in what it means about us when we accomplish or fail and how others might perceive us. "When you're not doing," he says, "everything you do exposes the light of truth."[6] In essence, with perfect action you are authentic and in the moment, and whatever happens is a direct result of your mindset.

You might be wondering how you can accomplish this art of non-doing. I will share two ways. The first is the essential practice of meditation. This is a tool that "trains the mind and reshapes the brain."[7] It's a continual practice of clearing your mind and going beyond your thoughts. When you direct this mindfulness to your actions, you can get in the zone, become one with the action, leave behind all judgments, get out of the way, and achieve perfection.

In 2017, Alex Honnold climbed El Capitan, a vertical rock formation of 2,900 feet at Yosemite National Park, without ropes and in under four hours. The *New York Times* referred to his climb as "one of the great athletic feats of any kind, ever."[8] What is so astonishing about this accomplishment is that most people would not even attempt it, let alone be successful. One misstep and you tumble to your death. This can easily bring up intense fear, which serves as a distraction. It seems Honnold was able to focus his mind, become one with the rock, and focus on where he was going rather than whether he might fall.

Your work may not be as treacherous, but it may bring up fear when you have to take risks. Develop "tremendous attention." With extreme abandon, avoid thoughts about success or failure, like "I'm going to flunk this" or "I'm going to ace this." These are future-based thoughts that take you out of the moment.

The second way to accomplish non-doing according to Samvara is that "when you are impeccable and selfless, there is power in everything you do."[9] Taking perfect action to help others rather than focusing on what success or failure means about you makes you more powerful and allows you to derive more meaning from your efforts.

According to the theory of karma, your intentions and good deeds today contribute to your future happiness. As the saying goes, "You get what you give."

HARD WORK AND SUCCESS

In chapter 2 we defined the term "high achiever" and saw that it applies to someone who works hard and succeeds. There are some truths to this definition and some myths to it as well.

Truths

To be successful, you need to work hard, but this is less about putting in endless hours, taking on copious amounts of work, or pushing yourself beyond a state of balance where your work interferes with your health and personal life. Hard work, as it is defined here, is about directing your mind and moving beyond self-judgments, fears, and the tendency to avoid. You are a high achiever when your mind is not cluttered and you can attend to the task, take action with "tremendous attention," and let go of any attachment to the outcome. This is associated with achievement because your perceptions affect your efforts. Your perceptions are how you focus. Your efforts are how you act. Your mind shapes your success.

Myths

This chapter has demonstrated that you can work hard and not have success. When you hold yourself back with your limiting beliefs, it leads you to sabotage your efforts. This can result from attempts to get too much done without mastering anything or being clouded by your thoughts so that you take less action. The fact that you are busy does not mean you are effective with your energy.

To be successful, all that is required is intention of mind, acting with attention, and removing thought. This eliminates the need to work as hard as you otherwise do and alleviates both the pressure of having a certain outcome or the attachment of meaning you assign to your self-worth. You can have perfect action without perfect results, but while the former will lead to success in the long run, the latter won't.

CONCLUSION

The demands of the workplace can certainly lead to burnout, but the demands you place on yourself can change your experience. You have more control over your mind and the quality of the effort you put forward than over your environment. Therefore, it is in your best interest to harness your power from within, to train your mind to work for you rather than against you, and to understand what leads to real success, not just moment to moment but also long-term.

Exercise for Step 6

If you've never intentionally tried manifestation, consider this a simple experiment. The following five steps are designed to help you focus your thoughts and intentions. In the final step we'll delve deeper into the concept of manifestation, exploring how it relates to the law of attraction, which suggests that by focusing on positive outcomes you can attract positive experiences into your life.

Step 1: Decide what it is you would like to manifest. It might be a raise, to connect to someone of influence, or to come up with your next big idea. Write down exactly what you want to see happen in specific detail.

_____

_____

_____

_____

Step 2: Create an affirmation about your vision coming to reality and write it down. If, for instance, you want an extra $5,000, say "I am experiencing increase right now. I favor $5,000 coming into my bank account."

_____

_____

_____

_____

Step 3: Practice your affirmation each morning when you wake up and each evening before you go to sleep. Keep your eyes closed as you would in meditation. As you say this phrase to yourself, visualize your desire manifesting as if you were watching a movie.

Step 4: As you meditate on this vision, ask questions about what you need to do to make it come true.

Step 5: Journal those questions and their answers. Any answers you receive to your posed questions are items on which you need to take action. Write these down and then go into immediate action mode.

_____

_____

_____

_____

Enlightenment

*You are not a drop in the ocean. You are
the entire ocean in a drop.*
RUMI, *THE ESSENTIAL RUMI*

Once you are managing yourself well, have your needs met, are
focused on getting things done, and have the right mindset in
place, this final step is about helping you create practices for
resilience. This entire book has been a buildup to this very moment, when you find out how to bring it all together and elevate
yourself to higher ground.

In discussing this step to burnout recovery, we will uncover
what enlightenment is all about, why it's essential, and what it
takes to reach it. I explain the importance of mindfulness and
meditation, among other positive practices.

CHAPTER 31

What Is Enlightenment?

Consider how you feel in your body when you are mentally and emotionally exhausted. There is a heaviness that makes it hard to get through the day. Your brain is in a whirl of cynicism and negativity. You feel hopeless about the possibility of change or that things can turn around.

In contrast, enlightenment is a lightening of your load. This occurs when you free yourself of the inner dialogue that brings you down and of the exhaustion you feel that impairs your ability to perform.

Enlightenment is something that happens as a result of training your brain to focus impeccably. It is the ultimate control that allows you to feel free and in charge no matter what you are facing.

Keep in mind that enlightenment is the result of advanced skills. That is why it is the final of the seven steps to overcoming burnout.

This does not mean you have to wait to start your brain training until you've mastered your emotions, empowered yourself, gotten to a state of flow, or watched your efficacy soar. Instead, it's a skill that you can start to develop alongside these other feats and increase the speed with which you experience success.

INNER RESOURCES

Much of what we discussed in the early part of this book is about external circumstances that lead to burnout, especially high demands and low autonomy. Remember, there will always be aspects outside of your control, but looking within can help you stay afloat.

We all experience some degree of stress, but what is it that enables some people to survive extremely stressful situations while others burn out? That is the question that medical sociologist Aaron Antonovsky wanted to answer. He researched Holocaust survivors to uncover the mystery. Antonovsky found that when people have a strong "sense of coherence" (SOC) about themselves and the world around them, they are more resilient.[1]

SOC is characterized by the confidence that you can make sense of your experience, that you have the resources to manage external demands, and that you can assign meaning to, and consequently become committed to, the challenges you face.

While your situation at work is by no means life or death, there are lessons to be learned about coping from this extreme example that can help prevent burnout. Because stress results from the perception that the demands exceed your resources, by challenging yourself to look for alternative and more positive interpretations of a difficult situation, you can increase efficacy and resilience. Your mind is designed to create a story around your experiences. So be aware of the story you are telling yourself and make sure that it is one that empowers you.

JOURNEY TO A MEANINGFUL LIFE

The journey toward a meaningful life is about using intention to guide your behaviors. It's about declaring what you want and going after it. And it's about seeing the big picture. You have to live in the present with an eye out for the future. You can always climb higher, but it's the road in front of you that determines your experience.

Traditional office work is no longer the norm. With the rise of remote and hybrid work, many professionals now have the flexibility to work from home, a coffee shop, or even a different country. While the traditional 9-to-5, in-office workday still exists for some, the future of work is increasingly diverse and adaptable. Whether you're part of a fully remote team, a hybrid workforce, or a traditional office environment, it's important to find ways to make your work meaningful and fulfilling.

The Holocaust survivors in Antonovsky's research created meaning of their dire circumstances, which allowed them to withstand extreme hardships. We arrive at meaning through the stories we tell ourselves so that we are resilient enough to cope with challenges. Therein lies the need to focus on perception.

Take a snapshot of your life. When you look back at the most difficult events you've endured, what impact have they had on you? Can you see patterns in how you've reacted during stressful times? And when you think ahead, knowing what you know about the way you've been handling stress, what concerns you the most?

It is said that it's not what happens to you that leads to stress, but your interpretation of what is happening. Your reaction is very much tied to your perception, which is associated with variables like your mindset, self-efficacy, sense of purpose, personal values, desire for control, coping style, personality, and recovery habits, to name a few. In short, your style of thinking, the way you feel about yourself, and your personal preferences lead you to process information in your own unique way.

If it's true that your interpretation of events is what matters the most, then your way of thinking about external events is your ticket to making dramatic and desired changes. And if you want to withstand stress, to manage your emotions well, and to create healthy habits that lead to success, you need to understand the psychology of the mind and its connection to your feelings and actions.

Picture yourself in a packed concert hall, surrounded by thousands of fellow music enthusiasts, all reveling in the joy of a shared passion. The atmosphere is electric, and you're thoroughly immersed in the experience. Then, without warning, the ground beneath you begins to tremble. The music screeches to an abrupt halt, and the realization hits you like a shockwave—you're in the midst of an earthquake.

In this moment of unexpected turmoil, each person in that concert hall is likely to react uniquely. Some, after the initial jolt of fear, may succumb to anxiety, their screams piercing the air. Others might opt to lie down, seeking a closer connection to the ground's vibrations, an attempt to fully embrace the surreal quake. For a few, despair may wash over them, as thoughts of impending doom and unsaid farewells fill their minds. It's a reminder that even in the most unexpected and unsettling moments, the human experience remains profoundly diverse and unpredictable.

Why is it that individuals sharing the same physical space and witnessing the same events emerge with vastly contrasting emotions and behaviors? As you've come to understand, these differing reactions are a product of the unique lenses through which people perceive the world, lenses crafted by their early life experiences. Consider this: In the case of parents' divorce, many children internalize it, believing they played a role in its occurrence. Similarly, when an adult raises their voice, children often internalize it as a reflection of their own inadequacy, convincing themselves that they are inherently flawed or insufficient.

In their young minds, a troubling narrative unfolds—the belief that if only they were smarter, funnier, thinner, or somehow "better" than they currently are, their parents would love them unconditionally, never raise their voices, and their lives would mirror the fairy tales they've read.

When we're young, we think we are the center of the universe. If anything happens, it's because of us. We don't yet have a concept of others. When mom raises her voice, we don't stop to think that maybe she's had a stressful day at work. When our peers don't want to share their newest toy with us, we believe it's because we're not cool enough.

Fast forward to adulthood. You are now old enough and experienced enough to understand that what happens to you is also a result of other factors outside of yourself. If you get in a fight with a friend, you may fault the friend, you may blame yourself, or you may consider how each of you contributed in a certain way.

Keeping this in mind can help you be more coherent in your thinking about yourself and others and lead you to mindfully interpret events in a way that boosts your inner resources rather than depletes them.

When all else fails, remind yourself that if meaning can be found in the Holocaust, it can be found anywhere when you search hard enough.

TABLE 31.1 Learning from Your Past

What are the three most difficult events or situations you've endured in your life so far?

1. _____

2. _____

3. _____

What impacts have these events or situations had on you?

1. _____

2. _____

3. _____

How did you react to each of these events or situations?

1. _____

2. _____

3. _____

What patterns do you see in your reaction to stressful events or situations?

_____

_____

Knowing what you know about the way you've been handling stress, what concerns you the most?

_____

_____

What can you apply from this book that can lead you to more optimal outcomes?

_____

_____

CONCLUSION

Enlightenment is an advanced skill that results from having ultimate control over your mind. By eliminating negative thinking, you lighten your load and can achieve outstanding outcomes without burning out. Having a strong SOC can help you be more resilient to the effects of stress. Acting with intention and a sense of purpose can increase your SOC and help you avoid the pitfalls of the mind.

CHAPTER 32

Why Enlightenment
Is Important

Enlightenment can do more than just help you survive highly stressful circumstances; it allows you to thrive as you create your reality. As a result, you can have peak experiences, live up to your full potential, and lead a purposeful life that brings fulfillment.

PEAK EXPERIENCES

When you follow the steps in this book, not only do you avoid burnout, you also learn how to function at an optimal level, which is known as a "peak experience." Such extraordinary moments are ones in which you feel profoundly alive, aware, and euphoric. These are also moments when you are simultaneously self-sufficient and integrated in the world, have a greater awareness of truth, and are living in harmony.

Recall that when you are in flow, time seems to slip away. You immerse yourself in the task to the point of losing track of time. Similarly, while having a peak experience, you are free of the confines of time and space; you are fully present and functioning to your fullest potential without effort or strain. Your fears and doubts vanish, allowing you to think flexibly and be creative.

SELF-ACTUALIZATION

Refer back to Maslow's hierarchy of needs (figure 4.1). The needs that correspond to the first four levels of the pyramid (physiology, safety, love and belonging, and esteem) are considered "deficit needs." When any of these needs remains unmet, it triggers a sense of deficit, propelling you to seek their fulfillment. However, once these fundamental needs are satisfied, they provide a sense of contentment but no longer serve as motivators to drive you toward realizing your full potential.

The ultimate goal, according to Maslow, is self-actualization. You reach the top of the pyramid when focusing on higher-level needs. In striving to always better yourself beyond the basic foundation, you create a state of harmony and understanding and realize your full potential. The values Maslow associated with this state include ones of integration, self-regulation, self-sufficiency, playfulness, effortlessness, and simplicity. In short, a balanced, happy, and easy life. It's what we all want deep inside, but what so few of us ever experience.[1]

CREATING A BALANCED LIFE

When people hear the word "balance," they automatically think about an even split between work and personal life. Given the demands of the workplace, this is impossible to achieve. But balance is not about an equal quantity between the two camps.

You already know that you have a whole slew of needs. When you focus on work, you may be taking care of your physiological, safety, and even esteem-related needs. But when work takes up too many of your resources, you end up not having the time to pursue meaningful relationships or the energy to take care of yourself properly.

I've heard many people say that although they know how important it is for them to exercise, for example, there just isn't enough time in the day. And even when there is time, they don't have the energy for it. On the surface, all these claims seem valid. But there is another way.

You know how when you really want something you find the time, the energy, or the money for it? A business coach I worked with once said that we all have resistance and make excuses. He used to share with prospective clients that if presented with an opportunity to buy a $100,000 car for only $70,000, they would somehow find the money. Why? Because they would see it as a deal they couldn't refuse. They could easily turn around and sell that car for an instant profit.

How can you think about your health and relationships as that profitable investment? Instead of thinking of the resources you're lacking, ask yourself how you can muster the energy, the time, and the money to do what you really want.

We often assume that having more time would lead to greater productivity, but this isn't always the case. Proximity, rather than time, can significantly impact our actions. For example, when I worked a hybrid schedule I was more likely to exercise on days I was in the office, even though I had more time at home. This is because my office was conveniently located near my gym.

How can you leverage the principle of proximity to accomplish your goals? Whether it's physical proximity to resources like your gym or digital proximity to mentors and high-performing colleagues, you have more control over your outcomes than you might realize. The key is to be strategic in your planning and creative in your approach.

When time seems scarce, it's crucial to prioritize. Start with what you want first and plan the rest of your life around those activities. For instance, if you want to join a meditation circle, find out when it's held and block that time in your calendar. For healthy eating, consider meal planning with quick, nutritious recipes that require minimal mental energy. To improve sleep, use technology to your advantage by setting bedtime alerts on your devices.

However, be mindful of how you allocate your energy. The rise of remote work has blurred the lines between personal and professional time, making it more important than ever to set clear boundaries. A recent study found that proximity to co-workers can increase long-term human capital development but may decrease short-term output.[2] This highlights the need for balance in our interactions and activities.

Consider the example of a client who found herself drained from constant socializing after work. By limiting social outings to two nights per week, she created space for rest and other opportunities, ultimately feeling more balanced and energized.

In today's hybrid work environment, it's crucial to be intentional about both physical and digital proximity. Evaluate what's consuming your resources outside of work. Are you spending too much time in virtual meetings? Are you able to create a productive home office environment? By creating boundaries around your time and strategically managing your proximity to resources and people, you can optimize your energy for the things that matter most to you.

Remember, the goal is not just to manage time, but to manage energy and proximity in ways that enhance both short-term productivity and long-term growth.

CREATING A HAPPY LIFE

Happiness: So much has been written on the subject. It is what we are all after, but we don't always go about it the right way. We seek immediate gratification because we don't want to wait to feel happy, but what greets us now doesn't always add up to joy. So how can you create a purposeful and happy life?

One of the regrets stated by the palliative patients mentioned in chapter 14 was that they wished they could have had the courage to be themselves. Are you living for someone else's happiness or your own? Do what makes you happy. Be authentic and listen to your inner voice.

Lastly, ask yourself, "How can I let myself be happier?" You may come up with some ideas but feel some resistance in pursuing them. If so, challenge the limiting beliefs that hold you back—beliefs that you don't deserve to feel happy, that it's not possible to have what you want, or that it is too scary to face change. Focus on how you will feel when you accomplish the items on your list and let the end result motivate you to take action.

CREATING AN EASY LIFE

"Easy" is a subjective term and can mean different things to different people. For our purposes, we are defining this word according to Maslow's definition, which includes "effortlessness" and "simplicity."

Imagine an experienced ice skater who expertly maneuvers around the rink, performing difficult moves that would knock an amateur off their feet in two seconds flat. The skater makes

TABLE 32.1 Cultivating Quality Relationships

If relationships are important for happiness, consider the
different relationships you have in your life. Who is in your
innermost circle? In the table below, rate the quality of your
closeness to those individuals on a 10-point scale (1 = low
quality, 10 = superior quality).

First-Tier Relationships	1–10 rating

How can you continue to foster those essential relationships,
whether with your spouse, your children, or your closest
confidant?

_____

_____

_____

Consider who is in your second- and third-tier circles.

Second-Tier Relationships	Third-Tier Relationships

- Are you investing your time and attention outside of work according to these tiers or do you need to rethink your paradigm?
- If you want to create new relationships, what are you doing about it?
- If you are seeking a romantic partner, are you out there dating?
- Are you investing energy in forming a community?
- Are you keeping in touch with old friends?
- Are you finding ways to spend quality time connecting to others outside of social media?

it look easy, and, in fact, it may be effortless for them if it is a peak experience and they are self-actualized.

The same is true for you. Surely there are tasks that you can do without much effort because of your expertise. But even more so than your experience, what leads to effortlessness is when you are working in a framework that allows you to reach optimal performance. This is when you are fully engaged in the work without distraction, when what you are focused on is meaningful or enjoyable, and when you are managing your energy to avoid depletion.

In *Barking Up the Wrong Tree*, author Eric Barker cites research that shows that people who relinquish unattainable goals feel happier and less stressed than those who keep working on such goals.[3] Exerting energy on impossible tasks prevents you from being in a state of effortlessness.

The other aspect of an easy life is when you employ simplicity in all that you do. What this refers to is monitoring your mind to ensure you aren't ruminating endlessly about your past mistakes or worrying about future ones. It's about letting your

---

TABLE 32.2 Overcoming Indecision

Indecision can happen as a result of incidents in which you learned it's not safe to make a wrong decision or have a less-than-perfect outcome. Follow these five steps to decide about an area where you find yourself to be indecisive:

1. Close your eyes and take a moment to ground yourself by taking several deep breaths.
2. Bring to mind an area of your life where you tend to be indecisive.
3. Tune into yourself. The truth behind this indecision is that you do know what you want, but you don't permit yourself to want it. Notice how this idea resonates in your body.
4. Consider the different options available to you and notice how they each resonate in your body.
5. Decide to go with the idea that resonates best with you.

---

intuition guide you rather than overthinking your decisions or overriding what feels right with what seems logically correct. You might think of simplicity as the result of designing and then living your life on purpose. It becomes as easy as plug and play.

CONCLUSION

Embracing enlightenment isn't just about getting through tough times—it's about thriving in them. When you dive into enlightenment, you unlock these incredible moments when life feels richer, where you're fully alive and buzzing with energy. It's like Maslow says: There's this ultimate level of self-realization waiting for us, where everything just clicks into place.

Finding balance isn't about splitting your time evenly between work and play. It's more about being smart with your energy and focusing on what really matters. Ever notice that when you really want something, you somehow make it happen? It's all about setting boundaries and making room for the stuff that makes you truly happy.

And speaking of happiness, it's all about being true to yourself. Forget about trying to fit into someone else's idea of what happiness looks like. Embrace your quirks, challenge those nagging doubts, and go after what lights you up inside. Keep things simple, too—less worrying about the past or stressing about the future, more going with your gut and living life on your own terms.

Rather than see enlightenment as some far-off goal, think of it as a journey, a constant process of growing, learning, and finding joy in the everyday.

CHAPTER 33

Living on Purpose

Sometimes making a living and making a life
point in opposite directions.
Pico Iyer, *The Art of Stillness*

Living on purpose refers to aligning your decisions with your values. To accomplish this you need to have self-awareness about what you deem valuable. That said, when it comes to work, there are certain values we can all agree upon. From my experience of coaching professionals on their careers over the past two decades, I've aggregated a dozen such values.

It seems that one of our dearest work-related values is *flexibility*. We want the ability to alter our schedules to meet the needs of life outside of work. If you have to see a doctor, you want to be able to make up the hours before or after your appointment. When you need to focus without distraction before a deadline, you want the ability to work from home so you can get more done. And when you are ready to go on vacation, you don't want your boss to say, "No, your coworker has already requested those days off," especially when you have a family event that is outside of your control.

As in any relationship, *trust* is a significant value. We all want to feel trusted, and, of course, we have to earn that trust. If you say you are working from home and are being productive, you don't want your manager to be suspicious of foul play. You also want to trust your manager. When you work as a unit and are outlining your goals for a promotion, you want your manager to provide feedback and help set you up for success rather than be passive-aggressive and skip your weekly meetings or cancel on you at the last minute. Trusting your coworkers is essential because you spend most of your time around them. You don't want to share something confidential with a teammate only to have that person tell their manager about it and have it come back to you. Lastly, you want to feel trust in the company you represent. If the company is either not following its stated values or if it is acting unethically, this can lead you to feel frustrated and even unsafe.

You want to feel the work you do serves a higher *purpose*. I've spoken with plenty of individuals who were unhappy with their job for any number of reasons. But one of the factors that made them hesitate to leave was that they really believed in the mission of the company. When a company's mission is aligned with your values, you feel like your work is meaningful and is serving the greater good.

While the top three values of flexibility, trust, and purpose are universal, there are many other values that you may want to home in on in your search for a meaningful career.

Values can be looked at as intrinsic if they are qualities that live inside of you and extrinsic if they are benefits from the job that affect your life.

INTRINSIC VALUES

Autonomy is an example of an intrinsic value. Most people I've worked with state that this is crucial to them, and given what we know about burnout, this makes sense. They want to be able to self-manage. They trust themselves to do a good job, don't

TABLE 33.1 Thinking Ahead

At the end of their lives, some people lament having worked "so hard" doing what they thought was important and missing opportunities to live full out. When you think ahead to your last days, how do you want to remember your life?

_____

_____

_____

Chances are you want to feel like you lived your life fully, that you felt loved by those around you, and that you left behind a legacy as a contribution to those who will live after you. So where can you be spending more of your time?

_____

_____

_____

Whom can you be investing in besides yourself?

_____

_____

_____

How can you implement more relaxation and self-care into your everyday routine so you don't burn out or end up living with regrets of your own?

_____

_____

_____

want their manager looking over their shoulder micromanaging their every step, and feel a sense of pride when they take on a project and see it through to its completion.

On the other hand, if you're an individual who struggles with self-induced structure, you may prefer less autonomy and more direction. You might really like routine rather than flying by the seat of your pants. In such a case, autonomy may be a less significant factor in your decision-making about a job.

Innovation and *creativity* are big factors to keep in mind when thinking about a career. If you're someone who feels stifled when told what to do and how to do it, you need to keep searching for a position that gives you the opportunities to experiment and create. This decision isn't limited solely to your individual role but extends to the organizational culture of your workplace. In hierarchical corporate environments, you might encounter barriers to infiltrating established bureaucracies, which can impact your ability to innovate freely. In addition, consider your team dynamics, assessing their receptivity to collaborative brainstorming, ego-less idea-sharing, and collective problem-solving. These values often drive individuals to explore self-employment, where they can champion their unique ideas, believing in their potential impact on the world.

What do you find valuable in the work that you do? What frustrates you about your job? When you turn your frustration into a value that isn't being met, you can identify the sources that can direct your search in a more meaningful direction.

EXTRINSIC VALUES

Extrinsic values encompass various factors such as *monetary compensation, job security, work-life balance, acknowledgment,*

leadership opportunities, and the prospect of *travel*. You've likely come across the age-old adage "Work to live, don't live to work." Essentially, this adage emphasizes that work serves as a means to an end—a means to finance the life you aspire to lead. While work can offer more than just financial rewards, the central message here is that money often plays a pivotal role in motivating our professional endeavors. This is often mirrored in the compensation you receive, reflecting your desire for fair remuneration commensurate with your education, your prior work experience, and your achievements in your role.

You also want to know that your job is not in limbo. When you work for a company that has big layoffs, even when your position is salvaged, those layoffs still create anxiety in you about the future security of your job. When you have a conflict with your direct manager or a coworker who is entrenched with the union, you feel scared that your job may not always be there for interpersonal reasons. A sense of *security*, both financial and in keeping your job, lets you focus on the work and not on whether it will be there tomorrow.

Referring back to the quote about working to live, you want to avoid having your job take over every waking moment. Today, more than ever there is an expectation for workers to get the job done no matter what. Even if it is unspoken, you know that if you don't clear your plate today, more work will continue to pile on tomorrow. To avoid feeling overwhelmed, you stay at the office later and later or attempt to get home to spend time with your family but then return to the computer and phone to work late into the night. Whatever hopes you had for personal care have taken a back seat due to the never-ending amount of work in front of you.

If you don't want to burn out, consider how and where you work. Are there ways you can get through tasks more effectively by delegating, setting boundaries, and avoiding distractions? If you are doing everything you can and still can't seem to dig yourself out from the demands of your job, perhaps you are in the wrong industry. Plenty of people are willing to forego *balance* because they value financial security or work status more. But if you're someone who is pining for more time to spend on yourself and your relationships, look for a career that gives you the lifestyle you desire.

When you work hard on a project, you want to be recognized. When someone else takes the credit, when the work you do goes unnoticed, or when your project gets shifted to someone else midway, you feel like the rug is being pulled out from under you. This can be disorienting, feel like an injustice, and lead you to feel angry and ignored. Whether it's at work or in your personal life, when you invest in something or someone you want to *feel appreciated*. It's a universal desire because we are wired for connection: We want to know that our efforts count.

Consider how you like to operate. Do you enjoy helping people carry out their mission, as in the case of an executive assistant, or do you want to lead teams and be in charge? *Leadership* is a significant value to consider because if you enjoy being in a position of influence and mentorship, you need to seek out such opportunities. And if it doesn't suit you, be sure to focus your efforts on a job that does not require you to lead.

Traveling the world may sound like a dream, but if you've ever traveled for work you know that it can be less glamorous than it seems. That said, if *travel* is one of your values you can bridge your personal and professional life passions. Flight attendants get to stop over in domestic and international destinations and spend their days off taking in the sights and sounds of a foreign city. Business executives use their flight time to get work done in preparation for a big meeting in a town hours away from home. Do you like traveling for work or do you prefer sticking to your local routine?

By now I hope you are considering your values and whether you are living a purposeful life. If there are values that are important to you that aren't being represented in your current scenario, don't despair. It is better to know what your values are and then design your life around them than to be oblivious and wonder why you are burning out. That said, you also want your values to align with each other.

WHEN VALUES AND CAREERS ARE MISALIGNED: A RECIPE FOR BURNOUT

High-demanding careers can lead to burnout due to grueling hours and high expectations that emanate from both the industry and the high achievers in those industries. What we need to examine, though, is why individuals are drawn to those careers and what can be done to prevent burnout.

Examining Values

As a coach, I often want to know about values. We all have them, but we're not always aware of how they drive us. We sometimes focus on a select few while we ignore the rest.

When we were playing M.A.S.H. as kids, we'd scribble down potential futures, including prestigious careers like doctor or lawyer. We likely didn't know much about any single profession but we knew what adults had drilled into our heads: Be a doctor or a lawyer. These were considered respectable jobs. It's what you did with your life if you were smart. There is prestige associated with these trajectories, not only for the work but for the journey taken to get there. Besides, once you made it, wads of cash would apparently start falling on you from the sky.

As kids, we knew money was highly regarded. You could use it to buy most things. Those with money had more options, and options are good to have. You never wanted to be the kid whose family didn't have money because you couldn't allow yourself all the luxuries of life that your friends got to experience. And if you grew up without being able to afford what everyone else could, you wanted to make sure this trend didn't continue for the rest of your life. For many there was an expectation to become accomplished—to make your parents proud.

Surely, everyone has a different reason for why they enter into the career of their choosing. But when we start the coaching process, we want clarity. And by focusing on values we get a better understanding of what drives the individual's decision-making process.

Two critical value-driven questions are: (1) What are the values that led you to pursue your career? And (2) Are these the same values that keep you there? Some people might go into a career with passion and idealism but then find that while it is soul-crushing, it is also lucrative. As much as they would like to make a career move, they sometimes feel lost. How else will they be able to support their lifestyle? Any other career would likely mean a serious pay cut. So while altruism may have gotten them there, money is the value that might keep them in the game.

What if your personal values don't align with the norms of your profession? During a recent interview, an attorney shed light on his experience as a junior lawyer. He was instructed that to advance to a partner position, he needed to accumulate 2,500 billable hours each year for a decade. This target translates to 48 billable hours per week, not accounting for the many additional hours he couldn't bill for. It's worth noting that this calculation assumes he never took any time off, which in reality is not feasible. When considering the need for vacation and nonbillable hours, the workload inflates significantly, creating an even more daunting picture. This prevalent culture places immense pressure on individuals to conform or risk being deemed "subpar."

A mismatch in values is one of the reasons professionals burn out. Take a long hard look at why you do what you do, and if it isn't working for you, consider alternatives. Yes, sometimes these changes will require a change in lifestyle, at least in the short term. But you have to look at what the cost is of staying in your profession.

Stress as a Result of Mismatched Jobs and Values

If you're burning out because of your values being out of sorts with your job, you are at risk of experiencing chronic stress and developing stress-related problems. This can negatively affect your health in many ways, including a greater risk for developing 41 different autoimmune diseases (e.g., hypothyroidism, rheumatoid arthritis, psoriasis).[1] Researchers reported that men who had diabetes, heart disease, or a history of stroke and who worked in highly demanding jobs in which they had little control over their workload were 68 percent more likely to experience premature death.[2]

Stress can also have cognitive effects. Have you ever experienced the feeling of having a racing mind, making it impossible to switch off? You lie in bed, attempting to sleep, but your thoughts are in overdrive. Your day replays in your mind and you worry about the tasks awaiting you the next morning. Anxious about forgetting something important, you find yourself endlessly rehearsing it mentally. As a result, you end up losing precious sleep. Ironically, the lack of sleep leads to additional symptoms such as irritability and difficulty concentrating, just when you need focus and productivity. This state is often described as experiencing "brain fog."

BALANCING YOUR VALUES

Values encompass different areas of your life. You have work-related values (autonomy, financial stability, or finding a sense of meaning), family-related values (spending quality time with loved ones, helping one another, and being a role model for your children), and health-related values (feeling good physically, being in control of your emotions and behaviors, and experiencing peace of mind).

As you can guess, focusing on the various areas of your life is vitally important: You don't have to limit yourself to just one area. When you limit yourself, you might experience great success there but fail in all the remaining areas. If you're looking for an accurate measure of success, it might entail living a more balanced life. This is why we delve into values for the various life areas.

While you have your personal values, your workplace has values of its own. In today's day and age, the way to get ahead is to work more. When you prioritize your family, it creates conflict. You can no longer rely on your boss to remind you to go home at the end of the day; it is your job to be mindful of your time and of your commitments and to make informed decisions that are value driven. Otherwise, you'll experience guilt for having a life outside of work. You might believe that you should be working even when you're at home.

If you're chasing a paycheck, reflect on what's beyond the money. Is it family life, serving the community, or being a good

TABLE 33.2 Finding Your True North

Balance may not be what you care about most. What would be even better is making a positive impact on the world. What gives you the highest purpose considering your values?

_____

_____

_____

_____

_____

friend? Remember that money is a means to an end. When you get too caught up in financial goals, you can forget that life is more than a contest and that you get the most value out of relationships, not material goods. You likely need less money than you think to live a happy and meaningful life. Money is a tool, but you have to be guided by a deeper vision of what that money can provide you with and be sure to live with integrity.

CONCLUSION

Living an enlightened life means experiencing life to its fullest. In this state you encounter peak moments of optimal functioning and achieve self-actualization by cultivating balance, happiness, and ease in your life. Enlightenment entails living with purpose, where your choices align harmoniously with your values. It involves transcending the mere pursuit of making a living and instead centers on the art of making life itself the ultimate purpose.

CHAPTER 34

How You Can Reach Enlightenment

*If I really want to change my life, I might best begin
by changing my mind.*

PICO IYER, *THE ART OF STILLNESS*

While enlightenment is often associated with spiritual awakening, in this context we're using the term to describe a state of heightened awareness and clarity. It's about optimizing your mental state to achieve peak performance and live a more fulfilling life. This brain state results from brain training and is necessary to living your best life. Now that you know what it's all about and have some buy-in, let's uncover how you can get the results you want.

As I alluded to earlier, your brain can lead you astray. It can create meaning where there is none, interpret situations as threatening when they are simply colored by your personal lens, and lead to stress and burnout when it is working against you.

To best understand how you can overcome problematic thinking patterns and other cognitive obstacles, let me share with you what it takes to get unstuck.

GETTING UNSTUCK

You've likely experienced moments of frustration, thinking, "I'm stuck in this cycle, no matter how hard I try to break free." This feeling arises when you find yourself repeatedly engaging in the same unproductive patterns, seemingly unable to escape them.

There's a term for this common phenomenon: "self-sabotage." The term itself can be unsettling, as it implies that you're undermining your own efforts. While this is indeed happening, it's essential to understand that self-sabotage often operates at an unconscious level. You are inadvertently hindering your progress, but it's not a deliberate or intentional act on your part.

So what causes you to sabotage yourself, and what can you do to overcome this so you can live the life you actually want?

Self-sabotage is when you have an internal conflict. There is a part of you that wants something (e.g., more money, a promotion, a better relationship), but there is another part of you focused on self-preservation.

In fact, there are three obstacles that we contend with when we are stuck:

1. *Negative self-beliefs.* These are core beliefs you hold about yourself, other people, and the world. They are typically constructed in childhood or early life and create the lens through which you interpret events happening currently.

If you think to yourself that nothing you do is ever good enough, chances are you also don't believe you are good enough. If you can't seem to find the time to engage in self-care, you likely deem yourself unworthy. And if you are working too hard to avoid making a mistake, you likely see yourself as a failure.

When you link your self-worth with your productivity, you worry that every mistake you make will translate into a catastrophe. It's like putting all your chips on one number at the roulette wheel rather than recognizing that, in reality, you have chips on multiple numbers, that people don't expect you to be perfect, and that they won't throw you out simply because you made one mistake.

2. *Fear.* When you have beliefs like "I am a loser" and are faced with a challenge that, if successfully overcome, can result in a promotion, you are immediately filled with a fear of failure. Your fears and your core beliefs go hand in hand.

TABLE 34.1 Identifying Negative Self-Beliefs

Negative self-beliefs directly affect how you feel and how you behave. You may not be aware of what is driving your behaviors, so work backward by looking at what you did, reflecting on why you did it, and which negative self-belief might be a fit.

Fill in the table below accordingly. In the "Negative Self-Belief" column, put A for "I am not enough," B for "I am unworthy," C for "I am unlovable," or if there is a different belief you hold, write it in yourself.

Sabotaging Behavior	Why You Did It	Negative Self-Belief

If you let money, status, benefits, or other people's ideas sway you into a job that is wrong for you, no matter how hard you try to avoid it, you are likely to experience burnout. You will more easily reach a state of exhaustion and feel too tired to engage in life outside of work. This might also be the case if you outgrow your job. Sometimes you keep yourself stuck in a situation solely due to the fear of what will happen if you leave. This requires a perspective shift so you can see your situation from a different angle and then come back to take inspired action. Have compassion for yourself and recognize that you can make an intuitive choice rather than a fear-based one.

Instead of succumbing to fear of the unknown, consider this analogy: Picture yourself strolling through a dense forest where numerous paths stretch before you, their destinations uncertain. In such a situation you must make a choice, selecting one of the paths without knowing where it leads. It's a leap of faith into uncertainty.

Your chosen path might eventually lead to an obstacle, forcing you to retrace your steps to the initial fork in the road where alternative paths await your exploration. With each encounter you acquire valuable insights. The next time you venture into the forest, you'll recall your previous journey, avoiding the path you first took and opting for the second. In this way, you are learning and growing from your mistakes, turning them into guiding beacons on your path of exploration.

If you have a goal and aren't doing anything about it because you're worried you'll be rejected or embarrassed, you are choosing to stay stuck in your current circumstances. Recognize the choices you are making and the ones you are overlooking.

Fears come in many flavors. In addition to a fear of failure and a fear of the unknown, the most common fears include a fear of missing out and a fear of picking the wrong thing. The latter is what is known as an *opportunity cost*, and due to this fear, you are less likely to commit yourself to anything new. It's a sign that you don't trust yourself to make the right decision. You might be thinking, "Even if I made a decision, it might be the wrong one." Fear is an indication that you are in a state of conflict. There is a part of you that wants to find enrichment and meaning and another part that is worried about the lack of security in making a decision that is not guaranteed to succeed.

Lastly, believing you are a failure sends a message to your brain that instills fear in you. When you are in this state, you might think that when you see evidence to the contrary, you'll change your belief, but it doesn't work that way. As Seth Godin put it, "Stop engaging with the false theory that the best way to stop feeling like a failure is to succeed."[1] You have to believe in

---

TABLE 34.2 **Applying Lessons Learned**

Take a look at your past challenges and failures. What lessons have you learned?

_____

_____

_____

Rather than letting past failures undermine your confidence, how can you use them as opportunities to grow and improve?

_____

_____

_____

If what you want is success, keep in mind that people who take more risks are more successful.

your potential first (or at least that you are willing to try) and then take action to ever really have a chance.

3. *Emotional triggers.* When past negative events aren't properly processed, you may find yourself feeling triggered by situations that in some way remind you of the original trauma. These triggers can feel overwhelming and lead to the belief that you'll never get rid of them. They can also lead to worries about tackling them again in the future.

Anxiety is your way of planning in advance so that you won't be surprised by what happens. If you struggle with anxiety, you likely spend time imagining possible catastrophes in your mind. It's like packing a suitcase for a trip you don't know you're going to take. The truth is, the majority of what you worry about never comes to fruition and focusing on the negative only robs you of the present moment.

The better solution is to be in the present at all times, believe in yourself enough to know that you can handle whatever comes your way, and follow your intuition.

MINDSET

Even when you know what to do, if you have a limiting belief, you either won't take action or you will end up sabotaging your efforts. To eliminate these inner obstacles, you must understand what your unconscious beliefs are.

You might be pondering, "How can I eliminate something I'm not even aware of?" That's an excellent question. I've already outlined two approaches to address this. First, introspection is key: Ask yourself why you behave in certain ways, scrutinize common beliefs that often pose challenges, and determine if any resonate with you. Second, confront your fears head-on and uncover the underlying beliefs driving them. Pose questions like, "What belief leads to this fear?"

For instance, let's consider a fear of change. What underlying belief fuels this fear? Perhaps it's the fear of failure, accompanied by the worry that taking a risk might lead to adverse outcomes. Or it could stem from the concern that your success might unsettle those around you, prompting you to downplay your achievements to maintain connections. Maybe deep down you harbor doubts about deserving better circumstances or achieving significant feats.

Perhaps you struggle with indecision. You have analysis paralysis when faced with too many choices. You wonder where to start, so you never take flight. Remember, you don't need a guarantee of future success; you just need to take it one step at a time. When you are in conversation with another person, you don't plan out every sentence you will say; you listen to what they are saying and bounce off of that in a natural rhythm. In the same way, focus on one action at a time and see where that takes you. Then you roll with what's in front of you. Trust yourself to find direction from within.

Your core beliefs develop early in life. One of the most common beliefs I've seen in my clients is the belief of personal inadequacy, which drives the focus on productivity. By ensuring that what you do is good enough, you get a temporary sense of relief. It's as if you hope your output will be an indication of your worth. The problem is, as soon as you finish working on Project A, you barely have any time to absorb your achievement— you are off to Project B. Hence, the unrelenting nature of this mindset and the propensity toward burnout. Remind yourself over and over that contrary to popular belief, your worth does not come from your work. It comes from your true nature. When you eliminate fear, you are more present and can allow your best work to come forth.

By understanding your beliefs and how they are or are not serving you, you can decide to change them. It might feel scary at first to do things differently, but as the saying goes, "If you always do what you always did, you will always get what you always got." Be bold. Be brave. Be you.

Do you ever tell yourself, "When I get a raise, then I'll be happy"? My client Sally worked in sales. During one of our sessions, she told me she wanted to close a deal she was working on but had tremendous anxiety because she knew the customer was looking at her competition. She told me, "If I close this deal, I will be happy."

I explained to Sally that she doesn't have to wait to feel happy. She can choose to feel it in this moment regardless of whether she closes the sale. I then asked her some follow-up questions. Here's what I learned: Sally had closed a sale earlier in the week. She felt happy for one hour afterward, but then became anxious again as her focus shifted to the next sale she needed to make.

Her closing rate was 25 percent, which meant that she was spending 100 percent of the time feeling anxious before closing any sale, then feeling disappointed 75 percent of the time when the sale didn't close, and even when she did close a sale her happiness lasted for only a very short time.

If your happiness depends on circumstance, you are fooling yourself. This is a deficit model, where nothing is ever enough. The phenomenon of desires not being met that leads you to chase after a substitute is known in Buddhism as "hungry ghosts."

Focusing on money when what you want is happiness is a form of procrastination. You have less control over how much your boss will pay you than you do over how you feel. When you focus on the aspect of your life over which you have less control, you are likely to be less successful, which will then fill you with shame and self-doubt. You need to focus on finding satisfaction in what is in front of you rather than always living for tomorrow. Don't put your happiness on hold. Find joy in every moment.

One of the ways to adopt an abundance model is by practicing gratitude. Being grateful for what you have (even your challenges, failures, and difficulties) increases energy, reduces anxiety, improves sleep, and creates feelings of social connection.

To make the transition from a deficit model to an abundance model of thinking, you just need to change your viewpoint. Instead of "I have failed," tell yourself, "I can learn from my mistakes." Instead of "This is too hard for me," say, "I won't know until I try." Rather than becoming defensive or finding fault with others and saying, "Their advice doesn't help me," be open to influence and think instead, "I will try those ideas out."

To set yourself up for success, you need to program your mind in the direction of your goals. Here are five effective strategies to program your mind in the right direction:

1. *Visualization*. Dedicate time each day to vividly imagine achieving your goals. Picture yourself engaging in the desired work, feeling fulfilled and invigorated. Envision yourself eagerly starting each day, brimming with enthusiasm for the tasks ahead.

2. *Affirmation*. Speak your goals into existence by affirming them aloud as if they've already been accomplished. For instance, declare, "I am a suc-

cessful chef, renowned for my innovative recipes and beloved by diners. My work brings me joy and allows me to lead a fulfilling life surrounded by loved ones."

3. *Share your goals.* Open up to supportive individuals in your life about your aspirations. By making your goals public, you hold yourself accountable and benefit from emotional support. Consider partnering with someone who shares similar ambitions, fostering mutual encouragement and accountability.

4. *Prioritize wisely.* Focus on tasks that contribute most directly to your goals. Avoid spreading yourself too thin by attempting to tackle everything at once. Recognize the importance of resting and recharging, knowing that sometimes stepping back is necessary for long-term progress.

5. *Practice self-compassion.* Embrace the inevitability of setbacks and imperfections in your journey. Be gentle with yourself and reject self-criticism or comparison. Understand that progress is gradual and nonlinear, and appreciate each step forward, however small.

Now that you know how to get unstuck and how to get your mind to work for you, in the next chapter we will dive into some practices you'll want to adopt into your daily life that can enlighten you.

CONCLUSION

Before you can attain an enlightened state, you need to remove any mindset barriers that keep you stuck. In particular, pay attention to negative beliefs you hold about yourself, to fears, and to emotional triggers, all of which create anxiety and take you out of the present moment. Instead, create an abundance mentality by focusing on gratitude, using power tools such as visualizations and mantras, obtaining social support, prioritizing your time wisely, and applying self-compassion.

CHAPTER 35

Integrating Enlightenment Practices

Steal, or still, the echo, so that you don't allow an event,
however unpleasant or momentous, to claim any more time
than it took for it to occur.
JOSEPH BRODSKY, *LESS THAN ONE*

The heart of *The Burnout Solution* is all about the practices that really make a difference. You've probably dipped your toes into some of them already, like mindfulness and meditation. But in this chapter, we're going to dive deeper into how they can help stop burnout in its tracks. We'll chat about how to actually make these practices part of your routine and how they all work together to keep you feeling balanced and fulfilled.

MINDFULNESS

Mindfulness is like a superpower that helps you stay in the moment. It's all about being aware of what's going on in your mind at any given time and gently guiding it back to the present. When you're mindful, you can spot when anxiety starts creeping in from worrying about the future or dwelling on the past, replaying mistakes or hardships. It's like hitting the reset button for your mind, bringing you back to the here and now.

When you can step back and observe your thoughts, you gain the power to steer them in a more positive direction.

Here are the main hurdles you might encounter on your journey to mindfulness:

1. *Autopilot mode*: Have you ever found yourself going through the motions without really thinking? That's autopilot. It happens when you're so used to doing something that you do it without even realizing. This can lead to mindless habits and even self-sabotage because many of our limiting beliefs operate under the radar.

2. *Dissociation*: When faced with overwhelming emotions, your mind might check out and focus on something else entirely. This can be a sign that something in your environment is triggering you emotionally.

3. *Habitual thinking*: Do you sometimes criticize yourself without even noticing? That's habitual thinking. It can keep you stuck in the past, replaying mistakes over and over again.

4. *Attachment*: We often get attached to how we think things should be, whether it's clinging to the past or worrying about the future. These attachments distract us from the present moment.

5. *Lack of training*: Like an untrained puppy, our minds tend to wander all over the place. Training your mind to stay present takes practice. Mindfulness is all about gently guiding your mind back to the present moment whenever it starts to stray.

Mastering mindfulness can unlock a whole host of benefits. It boosts self-awareness and self-management, crucial components of emotional intelligence (EQ). It helps you conserve energy and identify tasks that bring you joy and challenge. It also acts as an early warning system, alerting you when you need to recharge or when your efforts aren't yielding the rewards you deserve. As you'll soon discover, mindfulness is your secret weapon against burnout by countering its main contributors: high demands, low control/resources, and depleted energy levels.

Mindfulness and Demands

Stress is based on the perception that the demands exceed your resources. When you focus on meeting demand after demand without taking time to replenish your energy, you can burn out. Therefore, high demands, low resources, and low energy often come together for the perfect storm.

When your work places a lot of demands on you, it can feel stressful if you think you don't have adequate time to finish your tasks, if you don't believe you are capable given your skill level, or if you lack the mental energy to focus.

Mindfulness is being aware of where you stand and is the first step toward taking the right action. It helps you discern what your stuck points are and gain control over your body and mind. Because stress is based on perception, when you utilize tools that bring you into the present moment, you get out of future thinking and can change your current state.

Through mindfulness, you slow your mind down. It allows you to dig deeper than merely focusing only on the external demands, on your negative thoughts about being unable to accomplish them, or on the lack of confidence you feel inside. You start to witness your breath and feel your body. You become aware of what might be scary, and you can challenge your thoughts to ensure that they are accurate rather than fear based.

Through positive self-talk you can build up your resilience, remembering challenges from the past that you've overcome and changing your perception about what is possible. When you take the time to process information rather than react to it, you can assess whether the demands are solely external or whether you are adding your own demands for perfection. This can allow you to adjust your expectations so you feel capable and more sure of yourself. Even if you need to take a step back before taking a step forward, by mindfully engaging in every moment, you are listening to your inner voice and honoring yourself.

It is said that we often overestimate what we can accomplish in one year but underestimate what we can achieve in three years. From my experience, I believe that we overestimate what we can achieve in a day, and when we burn out, we underestimate what we can accomplish in that same period.

I've worked with plenty of high achievers who really struggle with managing their time. One big reason? They tend to underestimate how long things actually take. And hey, life throws curveballs, right? Like when you plan a 30-minute commute and end up stuck in traffic or hunting for a parking spot. It's the same with projects—you might need help from others or you're just not feeling as focused as you thought. So, here's my advice: Always give yourself more time than you think you need. It beats stressing out and rushing around. Plus, having a bit of extra time between tasks lets you recharge your batteries before diving into the next thing.

Part of self-awareness is being mindful of your strengths and weaknesses. If you are given a task you deem to be beyond your skill level, consider whether this is indeed the case or rather a fear response to potential failure. If you truly lack the necessary skill, decide whether you are going to focus on professional development to fill in the gap or whether you are going to communicate about the inappropriateness of the assignment given your current knowledge and experience.

You already know that enjoyment increases task engagement. While it may not be realistic to expect that every aspect of your job will feel enjoyable, you can focus on the elements of the task that feel more pleasurable. Consider what about the work that you are doing provides you with an inherent reward and zoom in on that aspect to alter your perception of the task.

Challenging your perceptions of yourself and what is possible is one part of job crafting. The other part is making decisions about how you conduct your work to make it more meaningful. Research conducted by University of Michigan professors points to four techniques that can help professionals in the service industry craft their job to have a more significant impact (figure 35.1).[1]

1. *Go beyond your job description*. Nurses can educate patients on health care, lawyers can recommend reading for legal protection, and administrative assistants can broaden their skill set.

2. *Tailor your services to your customers' needs*. Bookkeepers can act as financial therapists, chefs can adjust recipes for dietary restrictions, and therapists can tailor sessions based on client goals.

3. *Minimize negative customer interactions*. Developing communication skills helps, but avoiding unpleasant customers when possible can reduce burnout. Just as restaurants reserve the right to refuse service, you can consider similar strategies in your field.

4. *Choose meaningful work contexts*. Decide where to work based on the population you want to serve, whether it's a hospital, clinic, agency, university, or private practice.

Go beyond
the basics

Tailor your
services

Avoid draining
customers

Work in
meaningful contexts

FIGURE 35.1 Making service work meaningful. *Source*: Adam M. Grant et al., "Impact and the Art of Motivation Maintenance: The Effects of Contact with Beneficiaries on Persistence Behavior," *Organizational Behavior and Human Decision Processes* 103, no. 1 (2007): 53–67.

TABLE 35.1 Mindfully and Meaningfully Managing Work Demands

1. Is the task within your skill level? (Y/N) _____

   - If you answered yes, skip to question 2.
   - Is this a fear response? (Y/N) _____
   - If yes, focus on overcoming your fear.
   - If no, do you plan to expanding your skill set? (Y/N) ____
   - If yes, what resources do you need? _____
   - If no, ask to be given a more appropriate task.

2. Is the task pleasurable? (Y/N) _____

   - If yes, skip to question 3.
   - Identify one or more aspects of the job that is pleasurable or provides an inherent reward.

   _____

   _____

3. How can you go beyond your job's basic functions?

   _____

   _____

4. How can you tailor your services more to your customers or clients?

   _____

   _____

5. How can you minimize negative communication with customers or clients?

   _____

   _____

6. Is the context in which you work meaningful? (Y/N) _____

   - If yes, congratulations!
   - If no, what other contexts can you work in that would be more meaningful?

   _____

   _____

Crafting your job to align with your passions enhances your work experience, self-image, and resilience, reducing stress. Job crafting involves understanding your needs, desires, strengths, and weaknesses, which mindfulness helps increase awareness of.

Mindfulness and Control

When you deem a task to be stressful, you are evaluating your resourcefulness and stating that you fall short to meet the demands this task asks of you. Part of your framework in thinking about resources is your desire for control.

Throughout this book you have seen the topic of control come up again and again. Control is an essential aspect of how you see yourself in the workplace. It's the reason people become perfectionists and are self-critical and judgmental of others. Let's take a look behind the scenes of how you might seek to gain control in ways that are sabotaging your intentions and how mindfulness can help you become more aligned with what you truly want.

As you know, perfectionism entails putting a ton of pressure on yourself to perform above and beyond expectations. So why would anyone in their right mind put such pressure on themselves? This behavior is in response to fear. If you are perfect, you reason, no one can criticize you. The hope is that your performance will speak for itself. And if you are perfect, you can feel superior and even criticize others, which protects you from getting hurt. The problem is that needing a goal to be perfect is not only unattainable, therefore setting you up for failure, but that in the process of aiming so high, you burn out.

Also, the downside of taking a perfectionistic approach is that it leads to loneliness.

Joey is a classic perfectionist, but where did it all begin for him?

Well, growing up, Joey was in a big family where attention was scarce. With four siblings vying for the spotlight, he learned early on that being neat and orderly was his ticket to standing out. It was his way of creating some sense of control amid the chaos.

Fast forward to adulthood, Joey's environment changed but his perfectionist tendencies stuck around. Now he's got a good job, a partner named Jenny, and a fear of not measuring up. He's always pushing himself to prove he's diligent, fearing that laziness might rear its head if he lets up for a moment.

Some days, Joey's riding high. When he nails his goals at work, he feels like he's on top of the world, strutting around with a sense of accomplishment. But when he falls short it's a different story. He beats himself up, feeling like he's not good enough.

Over time, this fear of failure takes hold. Joey starts procrastinating on tasks, convincing himself that if things don't go well he can blame it on not trying hard enough. But deep down he knows it's not true. And when failure does come knocking, it just feeds into his belief that he's not worthy.

So what does Joey do? He sets even higher standards for himself, hoping it'll finally silence that nagging voice of doubt. But the fear lingers, and the cycle of failure and avoidance keeps on spinning.

Perfectionism is an overcompensation for a sense of helplessness and is an attempt to find control. If the end result is that you feel worse about yourself because you've failed or exhausted yourself trying, you must find a better way. Ask yourself, "What would it be like to strive for excellence instead?" By taking your standards down a notch so that they are attainable and still very respectable, you have an opportunity to shine.

Rather than focusing on being perfect, aim to create a balance between doing good work and getting the job done. All too often you might find yourself lagging because the outcome of what you are working on doesn't meet your standards. The goal is to get it done well and move on. You have other fish to fry, so don't get stuck on just one fish. Once you finish your task, take time to appreciate your efforts and to be happy with the outcome. In other words, don't focus too much on what other people might think of it. Instead, give yourself a seal of approval.

By incorporating self-compassion, reframing failures, and giving yourself credit for trying even when what you tried did not come out as well as you would have liked, you can overcome perfectionism and engage in your work in a way that allows you to stay in the game long term and feel satisfied.

The good news is that by letting go of perfectionism, you will not only feel more satisfied in your work, but your relationships will benefit as well. According to one study, perfectionists were 33 percent less likely to have satisfying relationships.[2]

To help your relationships at the office and beyond, give yourself permission not to know all the answers. Admit your mistakes and take responsibility for your failures. Let go of excuses and rationalizations. Don't become defensive when someone points out something that bothers them about you or your work. Take a deep breath and remind yourself that you are enough and that as a human you aren't going to get it right all of the time. By reaching beyond your insecurities and opening yourself up to others, you can lead a more fulfilling life filled with connection rather than isolation.

As you've seen, the opposite of perfectionism is compassion. When you drop your critical self-statements and focus instead on self-assurance and on developing a growth mindset, you will feel better connected to yourself. This approach also provides you an opportunity to expand relationships with others, which, as we know, is what's most important in life at the end of the day.

Getting back to the issue of control, you want to seek control in healthy ways. True control comes from controlling your energy, your emotions, and your behaviors, which come primarily from being mindful. This means focusing on creating conditions that lead to optimal performance and letting go of any attachment to the end result. As Seth Godin says, "You're responsible for what you do, but you don't have authority and control over the outcome."[3]

In an attempt to be in control, you might try to control your feelings by fixing them, avoiding them, or distracting yourself—anything in order not to feel them. These approaches only lead your emotions to intensify. Even when you're not aware of your feelings, if they are left unprocessed they live in your body. Ultimately, you feel less in control by avoiding your feelings than you would be facing them. Only when you are mindful of your emotions and can self-regulate are you truly in control and can live without constant fear. Remaining unaware of how disconnected you are from yourself can lead to dysregulation, disorder, and disease.

When you have good self-management, you can engage purposefully in your work and feel satisfied. In *Why We Work*, Barry Schwartz explains this notion. He correlates work satisfaction with engagement, challenge, autonomy, and "making a difference in the world."[4]

If you tend to focus a lot of your energy on what other people might think about you, you are, in essence, giving away your power. You might let other people's perceptions of you sway your decisions, but this is a fruitless endeavor. You cannot control how other people see you, and rarely can you truly know what they are thinking anyway. Be mindful of what you are focusing on and why.

Joey would benefit from understanding that his perfectionism was born as a way of coping when his environment was chaotic, but that it's no longer serving him. Instead of tying his self-worth to his productivity, he should work on the belief that he is good enough just the way he is without any qualifiers. Instead of setting himself up for failure by creating unattainable goals, Joey would benefit from creating goals he could accomplish given his time, qualifications, and everything else on his

---

TABLE 35.2 Mindfully Attaining Control at Work

Put a check mark (✓) next to each strategy you are already using and an asterisk (*) next to the rest.

- ☐ Strive for excellent rather than perfect work.
- ☐ Balance doing good work and getting the job done.
- ☐ Appreciate your efforts no matter the outcome.
- ☐ Substitute self-assurance and a growth mindset for self-critical statements.
- ☐ Give yourself permission not to know all the answers.
- ☐ Admit your mistakes.
- ☐ Take responsibility for failures.
- ☐ Let go of excuses and rationalizations.
- ☐ Remind yourself that you are enough.
- ☐ Focus on what you can learn from each situation.
- ☐ Restrain yourself from focusing on other people's perceptions of you.
- ☐ Create attainable goals.

Consider incorporating items with an asterisk into your routine.

plate. By practicing self-compassion, he could stop being so hard on himself and thereby increase his motivation to work on his goals without fearing failure as much. But when he does experience failure, Joey could reframe it to mean that he is trying and learning along the way. He could give himself credit for his efforts and progress in his goals, no matter the immediate outcome.

By implementing the above changes, you, like Joey, could enjoy your work more. You would have less internal pressure to succeed and fewer harmful self-judgments and be more aligned with your goals. You would like yourself more and feel more comfortable sharing your talents with the world.

Mindfulness at Work

Mindfulness has been shown to decrease stress and anxiety, improve physical health, and increase EQ. Many companies are providing mindfulness classes to their employees and even starting their meetings with a meditation.

In *Mindful Work*, David Gelles cites findings from a study done at the American insurance company Aetna. There are high monetary costs to companies when their workers are stressed. To be accurate, Aetna found that it costs approximately $2,000 more per year in healthcare for each employee who was highly stressed. In 2012, Aetna began implementing mindfulness programs and found that their healthcare costs went down by 7 percent, the equivalent of over $6 million. And to put the icing on the cake, productivity went up by about $3,000 per employee. No wonder companies like Apple, Google, Intel, and many more are taking notice and implementing their own workplace mindfulness practices.[5]

According to the *Fiscal Times*, 80 percent of executives at General Mills reported being able to "make better decisions," and

89 percent "said they became better listeners" after practicing mindfulness for seven weeks.[6]

Findings from internal research done at the legal firm Herbert Smith Freehills point to a 10 percent improvement in employee performance after a six-week meditation program due to increased focus, efficiency, communication skills, and work-life balance.[7]

Clearly, mindfulness is beneficial mentally, emotionally, and physically. That said, let's see how to optimize mindfulness further.

MEDITATION

Mindfulness results from training your mind to be still. To attain such control over yourself, you need a tool. Meditation is just what the doctor ordered.

Throughout this book we've touched on meditation. You may have tried it in a yoga class or even adopted it as a practice. Whatever your understanding of this concept at this juncture, adopt a "Beginner's Mind"—approach meditation with fresh eyes and an open heart.

There are many forms of meditation, so not all meditation is created equal. We could argue that any kind of meditation is beneficial but you need to properly align your goals with your tools to have the desired results.

Meditation can be guided or unguided. The beauty of guided meditation is that it is sometimes easier to keep your mind focused this way, and it's an excellent way for beginners to get acquainted with the nature of their mind.

Guided meditations can be used for relaxation, to increase awareness of bodily sensations, to connect you to spirit, to boost empathy for others, and to help you visualize something beyond what you usually allow yourself to consider possible.

These are all wonderful ways to get into a positive space, but they don't necessarily train your brain to increase mindfulness. There is a meditation practice dedicated to this particular skill. If you want to increase your mindfulness muscle, practice a mindfulness-based meditation.

Your mind produces thousands of thoughts each day, and if you let it, ideas will endlessly stream in and out of your mind. The point of mindfulness meditation is to notice those thoughts rather than be swept up by them.

Imagine that you are a lifeguard. You are not in the water but rather watching the actions of those below you. Similarly, when you are mindful, you are the observer of your thoughts. This is the first step. Once you notice thoughts taking up space in your mind, you consciously let them go. The goal is to focus on the space between the thoughts and, over time, to increase that space more and more.

Once you have accomplished this feat in meditation, you can start applying mindfulness outside of the practice. When you are going about your day at work, you can begin to notice your thoughts and refocus your mind. You can be more aware of what would typically distract you and bring yourself back to your work. You can notice more keenly how you feel when you are interacting with others around you and keep your emotions in check.

If you want to be muscular, you will have to pump iron regularly to maintain your results. Going to the gym once or twice will not suffice. Similarly, meditation is a practice. In order to maintain its benefits, you will need to develop a routine around it. Even if it's only for five minutes a day, this is an opportunity for you to be consistent.

In *Altered Traits*, Daniel Goldman and Richard Davidson report on the changes to the brain that occur shortly after participants started practicing meditation. They found that the part of the brain where we process emotion (the amygdala) shows less reactivity to stress when people meditate. Also, participants' attention improved with practice. They were able to focus for more extended periods of time, their mind would wander less, and they improved their working memory, which allowed them to remember relevant information mid-task.[8]

To create an optimal meditation practice, focus on clearing out any clutter in your environment. Clutter blocks energy from flowing. If you've ever cleaned out your closet, you know how light you feel when there are fewer items around.

In addition to clearing physical clutter, make sure your financial affairs are in order. Pay off any outstanding bills. Focus on getting rid of any debts so you can feel financially free. Because

---

TABLE 35.3 Setting Yourself Up for Successful Meditation

- Declutter a space in your home for meditation so that you can create a peaceful and calming environment for your practice.
- Get your financial affairs in order so that you can reduce stress and anxiety, allowing you to focus on your meditation practice.
- Create a daily routine of meditating.
- Keep track of your meditation sessions manually or through an app (e.g., Insight Timer).
- Focus on the space between your thoughts.
- Each time you notice that your mind has wandered, bring it back without judgment.

money is energy, by eliminating debt you can attract more money into your life and have a stronger meditation as the energy flow is improved.

By stilling your body and staying consistent with your breathing, you can focus your mind and reach the calm you seek, the peace you crave, and the joy you desire. You may have to mourn your losses, resolve your grief, and overcome your anger and disappointments to get there, but happiness is always in the heart beyond these emotions. Access the visual guide to a mindfulness meditation at www.BurnoutToResilience.com.

SELFLESSNESS

Meditation offers a powerful tool for transcending the limitations of the ego. By quieting the mind, we can begin to unravel the layers of self-imposed beliefs and conditioning that often hold us back. This process of self-transcendence, or selflessness, involves moving beyond our individual identities and connecting with something larger than ourselves. When we let go of our ego-driven desires and attachments, we can experience a profound sense of freedom and clarity.

Our beliefs about ourselves and what is possible are often deeply intertwined with our personal histories. For instance, if you were raised to believe that you don't matter, you might interpret workplace situations as affirmations of your unimportance. When we carry these outdated beliefs into our current circumstances, we perpetuate self-sabotaging patterns that hinder our growth and fulfillment.

Recognizing these patterns is the first step toward breaking free. Through meditation and mindfulness, we can cultivate awareness of our thoughts and feelings, allowing us to challenge and reshape the narratives that no longer serve us. In doing so, we create space for new possibilities and a more authentic expression of who we truly are.

The self is also full of notions of how you compare to others. Often, this is how we decide about our self-importance. This can lead to arrogance on the one hand or a sense of insignificance on the other. When you derive your sense of self from what other people achieve or think, you are not only giving away your power but are more likely to engage in actions that you hope will gain you approval.

Your beliefs fuel your thoughts, which may leave you wondering, "How can I know if my inner voices are real?" They are a part of your experience, but are they part of the "self"? The keys to knowing your truth are to relinquish your need for admiration from others, follow your intuition, and listen to your body. Does the message you hear in your head resonate as truth or is it a reaction to a circumstance or an embedded sense of insecurity?

Meditation helps you gain clarity and erase the self. It is your chance to take a step back and separate what you're bringing in from your personal history and what is coming from the job. It is a reminder to give others the benefit of the doubt rather than letting your generalized distrust of people get in the way. By letting go of the self, you can have honest conversations and get the perspective of someone who has been in the company longer or who has more experience to widen your lens.

Erasing the self means letting go of the stories you tell yourself about yourself and others. It's about mindfully identifying where your fears and desires lie and letting go of your attachments to them. If you are afraid to go against the grain because of what other people might think, release this fear. If you aspire to get recognition for your work, without which you feel resentful, this is a desire to let go of. Fears and desires only bring suffering. By practicing selflessness you can be present and employ critical thinking rather than act impulsively, automatically, and mindlessly.

When you focus on desires, it brings up the fear of failure and the fear of missing out with worries such as "What if I don't get this?" Should you be successful in attaining your goal, you might become fearful of losing it and wonder, "What if I can't hold onto what I've learned?" or "What will happen to my newfound success if I make a mistake moving forward?" Focusing on all of these "what if" scenarios takes you out of the present moment so that you miss what is right in front of you. Instead of enjoying what you've accomplished, you're focused on potential disasters.

Take a step back to examine this pattern. From afar you can see that it is not rational. If you were to live your life like this, you would never do anything. You would never get married because of the fear of divorce. You would never go to school because you might not pass an exam. You would never venture abroad because you might not find your way. This is the true form of missing out.

In meditation, notice your thoughts and whether they are tied to fear or desire and let them go. Remind yourself that you want to live in the here and now so you can appreciate life more fully and feel fulfilled by what is currently within rather than what might be without.

While meditation provides a dedicated space for self-reflection and letting go, we can also cultivate selflessness in our daily lives. By focusing on the needs of others and the collective good, we can transcend our ego-driven desires and experiences a deeper sense of fulfillment.

For example, when my kids rush into the kitchen eager to help, they're not always thinking about making my life easier.

They're excited about the idea of doing something fun. If I ask them to do a simple chore like setting the table instead, they might grumble about it.

As a parent, I can lead by example by giving them a task that might not be as thrilling but still keeps them engaged. And when they willingly tackle less-exciting tasks just to lend a hand, that's when I know they're truly being selfless.

Being selfless is about wanting to do something that is not for yourself. Karma yoga is dedicated to making your work a spiritual practice whereby you selflessly give of yourself to your employer. Through this practice you derive a sense of purpose beyond your desires. It's about making a contribution; it's about having an impact that is not about you.

In a recent study, researchers examined how kindness relates to goal attainment.[9] Because altruistic kindness is associated with intrinsic rewards and the emotional part of the brain, when participants gave altruistically without any external reward, they reaped the benefit of their action immediately. Their prize was intrinsic satisfaction. When participants exercised strategic kindness, there was a delay in reward because this type of kindness correlates with extrinsic rewards. In other words, even when you are giving, if you are focused on what you will get in return, you will have to wait and see whether your actions get reciprocated or your reputation improves. But when you are selfless (or what these researchers referred to as "prosocial"), you end up with a greater reward because goal attainment starts immediately.[10]

By focusing on others, you tap into your giving spirit and thereby feel more connected. Your efforts have more significant meaning, which makes them more personally rewarding.

Sunshine was someone who worked in a deadline-driven environment. She would focus on getting as much done as she could before her deadline. Sometimes, however, she found that even with her most considerable efforts, she would not meet specific markers in time. Instead of wasting time and energy trying anyway, she would help her coworkers get more accomplished in time for their deadlines. Because she was generous with others, they would want to reciprocate the following quarter, which helped her reach greater heights than had she tried to accomplish her tasks alone. Not only that, she was well liked, and this made her working environment more pleasant and helped her feel easily motivated to go to work each day.

When you embrace selflessness, even during those marathon workdays, you don't feel depleted. It's like how being fully engaged keeps you going without exhausting you. Being selfless brings a similar sense of lightness. That's because shedding the weight of "self" makes everything feel lighter and more effortless.

Self-description holds you back. It tells you what you can and cannot do and is based on what you've learned from others. It's an illusion that makes you struggle and lose personal power. Release your personal history and self-description and find new possibilities within you.

When you immerse yourself in a task without the self, you go beyond thoughts and fears. You are pure action and allow intuition to guide you. This is a way to remain powerful.

Sometimes we think we have to do something to get to the next level. Enlightenment, which is the ultimate state of power, comes from doing nothing. By stilling the mind you gain self-control, can shed the self, and be fully present.

Consider yourself a selfless warrior who can stop thought in meditation and stop any attack against you outside of meditation through the purity of your mind.

TABLE 35.4 **Cultivating Selflessness**

Use meditation as a means to go beyond the self. Identify one item at a time from the list below you want to release and focus on letting it go in your meditation:

☐ Admiration from others
☐ Stories about yourself
☐ Stories about others
☐ Fears
☐ Desires

Use these guidelines to maximize your practice:

☐ Distinguish what is internal and what is external.
☐ Give others the benefit of the doubt.
☐ Employ critical thinking rather than acting impulsively, automatically, and mindlessly.
☐ Focus on the greater good rather than on your ego.
☐ Make your work a spiritual practice.
☐ Practice altruistic kindness without any external reward.
☐ Allow your intuition to guide you.

When someone else gets the promotion or attention you were seeking, be happy for them rather than bask in negativity about yourself.

Practice humility. Honor your opportunities. Take on new challenges, including delving into tasks that you don't like or are afraid of. This promotes growth and lets you reconstruct your story to be more fitting for where you are in that moment rather than staying stuck with the story of who you were.

HEARTFULNESS

Mindfulness is a way of gaining control over your inner world, and hopefully by now you see the benefits of practicing meditation and staying present. That said, there is a way to level up from there.

When you are mindful, you are focused on your thoughts. This is a good practice, as mentioned, but to be great you will need to focus on the heart.

Heartfulness goes beyond conscious awareness. It's what leads you to be free because it's not about just observing what is happening but rather about liberating you from limitation.

We saw how selflessness frees you from the confines of the ego, including fears and desires that ultimately lead to suffering. In a similar vein, heartfulness leads to transformation. It goes beyond your thoughts and into a deeper dimension that encompasses your values and true nature. When you are coming from the heart, you have compassion and a more positive frame of mind. On a day when you are struggling with work, heartfulness would allow you to take a step back and consider everything going on in your life. You could slow down rather than rush through every moment. This would center you with a greater appreciation for what you have.

Hamdi Ulukaya, the founder of America's biggest-selling Greek yogurt, Chobani, exemplifies heartfulness. It all started when he went to see a yogurt factory that had been in existence for 80 years and was closing its doors. He saw how the workers whose families had been at the factory for generations were being given up on and became upset by this. He decided to purchase the factory, rehire all the employees, and rebuild.

What made Ulukaya successful was his focus on community. He did not focus on the return on investment and how much money he could make. Instead, he focused on the people. He brought his heart into every decision, from training unskilled workers to employing refugees and immigrants in need of jobs. He focused on creating a thriving community with schools and soccer fields, and in return his company became wildly successful.[11]

Heartfulness is also about control and acceptance. Control is all about being on top of things, like knowing where your keys are or keeping your toothbrush handy on the bathroom counter. It's about setting up systems that make life easier so you're not scrambling around in a panic.

TABLE 35.5   Cultivating Heartfulness

Take a moment to recall what your intentions and vision for your career were when you first got started and write about this below.

_____

_____

_____

Now reflect on the person you have become since then.

_____

_____

_____

What changes would you like to make to realign yourself with the person you want to be?

_____

_____

_____

Acceptance is like shrugging your shoulders and saying, "It is what it is." Instead of stressing over things you can't change, like the weather or traffic, you roll with the punches and focus on what you can control.

When you mix control and acceptance together, you get a winning combo. You're more chill, more effective, and better able to handle whatever life throws your way. It's like having a secret superpower that keeps you calm and collected, even when things get crazy.

CONCLUSION

When it comes to beating burnout, there is no one-size-fits-all solution, but there are some key skills and ways of thinking that can transform your experience.

Your mind is key to this transformation because it is what brings about limitation. To conquer the mind you need to establish and maintain a practice of mindfulness through meditation. You need to move beyond the ego to overcome fears and desires so you can be more in the moment. Ultimately, you want to bring your heart into everything you do because it establishes a connection from which you will derive meaning and pleasure.

You have the power to design your life, to live with purpose and intentionality so that at the end of your days you can reflect back and feel contented and fulfilled.

Success comes in many forms. You have to reach beyond the materialistic world to find meaning. You find success when you are living authentically, when you can attain what you want beyond your basic needs, and when you surround yourself with other people. Take the advice of Albert Einstein: "Try not to become a man of success but rather try to become a man of value.

He is considered successful in our day who gets more out of life than he puts in. But a man of value will give more than he receives."[12] The real reward is about who you become in the process.

When you are aware of something that is not uplifting you, it is an energy drain. You then have an opportunity to fix it. Rather than focusing on the problem, utilize your tools of meditation, mindfulness, compassion, selflessness, and heartfulness to make things better.

Instead of waiting for the perfect circumstance to present itself to you, focus on finding perfection in every condition.

Even when you have the best plan in the world and the greatest strategy to help you implement it, you can get stuck. Ironically enough, you are the reason for this "stuckness." You get in your own way.

You do this by second-guessing your decisions, by going for instant gratification rather than thinking long term, and by letting your past determine your future.

Enlightenment is going beyond the limitations of your mind based on your personal history and tapping instead into your limitless potential. By letting go of your attachments to the past, you free yourself to explore what is possible, attain greater heights, and lighten the load you carry. Just decide to be positive in the face of negativity and you will be more powerful and experience more joy.

Exercise for Step 7

While the empowerment blueprint is engagement, the enlightenment blueprint is nonengagement, or keeping still. Some study participants who practiced meditation experienced improvement in focus and working memory after only two weeks.[1]

Now it's your turn. Over the next two weeks, set aside at least 10 minutes each day for some silent meditation. It's best to do this right in the morning, before you dive into your phone messages or email. Once you've gotten up, maybe had a shower and a glass of water, find a quiet spot, set a timer, and close your eyes. Try to clear your mind and focus. If your thoughts start to wander (which they probably will), gently bring your focus back without getting judgmental. The more you practice reining in your wandering mind, the stronger your mindfulness muscle will become. You've got this!

Fill in a daily entry for your start and end time as well as any observations about the practice itself (e.g., "I was able to bring my mind back twice today" or "I became aware of a pain in my body I didn't realize was there before").

Day	Start Time	End Time	Observations
1			
2			
3			
4			
5			
6			
7			
8			
9			
10			
11			
12			
13			
14			

Write below what changes you notice in your focus and working memory at the end of this two-week trial.

_____

_____

_____

_____

_____

If you found this helpful, consider maintaining meditation as a long-term practice.

Conclusion

From Burned Out to Fired Up

I walk down the street. There is a deep hole in the sidewalk. I fall in. I am lost. I am helpless. It isn't my fault. It takes forever to find a way out. I walk down the same street. There is a deep hole in the sidewalk. I pretend I don't see it. I fall in again. I can't believe I'm in the same place, but it's still not my fault. It still takes a long time getting out. I walk down the street. There is a deep hole in the sidewalk. I see it is there, but I still fall in. It's a habit. My eyes are open. I know where I am. It is my fault. I get out immediately. I walk down the same street. There is a deep hole in the sidewalk. I walk around it. I walk down a different street.

Portia Nelson, *There's a Hole in My Sidewalk*

THE SEVEN-STEP BURNOUT SOLUTION

If you've been going through life in the same way and getting the same results, it is time to take responsibility and find a new way. This book provides you with a seven-step solution to burnout, each of which contains scores of additional resources and ideas. All the information you need about how to approach your circumstances differently is here. Now it's time to implement it.

People burn out for different reasons depending on varying levels of demands and control, so it is necessary to start by identifying where you are on the engagement spectrum. To shift to optimal engagement and attain optimal performance you'll need to take seven steps.

Step 1: Enhance your emotional intelligence (EQ) by understanding your needs and upgrading your self-talk. Recognize your strengths and learn to control your emotions effectively.

Step 2: Empower yourself by prioritizing tasks and eliminating distractions. Recognize what gives you power and what takes it away, empowering yourself to face challenges with determination.

Step 3: Dive into tasks you've prioritized for optimal engagement. Enjoy your work without feeling overwhelmed. Strive to be fully immersed without drowning in tasks.

To perform optimally, fulfill your need for autonomy. Even if you can't make every decision, embrace the mindset that you choose your actions. Don't see yourself as a victim of tasks; acknowledge your choice in every moment. Remember, you always have the power to choose differently.

Enhance engagement by accessing job and personal resources like social support, hope, efficacy, resilience, and optimism. Develop strong time management skills to be efficient and effective. Identify obstacles to optimal engagement and focus on bolstering your inner resources.

Step 4: As you engage in tasks, celebrate your accomplishments. Reflect on them to boost your efficacy. Recognizing your achievements builds confidence and pride, empowering you to take on new challenges. This confidence fuels your courage to pursue even greater endeavors over time.

This is the action-focused protocol. However, to go higher, feel more fulfilled, live up to your potential, have a sense of purpose, and live the life you want to live, you need to incorporate three additional steps.

Step 5: While you're busy with tasks, it's crucial to monitor your energy levels to ensure you have enough fuel to keep going. Take breaks during the workday and plan periodic vacations to recharge. Remember, your worth isn't defined by how hard you work or others' perceptions of you. Quality work matters more than hours clocked in. If you feel drained, prioritize self-care to replenish your energy. Setting boundaries and valuing yourself beyond productivity are key.

Step 6: Use your energy wisely by engaging in work that aligns with your motivations. If you're solely focused on external rewards, it might indicate that the job isn't the right fit. While recognition and fair pay are important, seeking intrinsic rewards like a sense of purpose can be more fulfilling. Instead of justifying staying in a job you dislike with raises or promotions, focus on finding satisfaction in meaningful work. Also, consider the power of manifestation to attract what you desire, making your efforts feel more effortless.

Step 7: The final step in your burnout recovery journey is enlightenment. I define this as getting the right mindset so you can lighten your mental load. This happens through a training of the mind, using meditation and mindfulness practices.

Enlightenment is also about living a balanced life through selflessness and heartfulness. Rather than having your work burn you out, you need to have a burning ambition to engage in your work for the sake of the work itself, not for the results it will yield. When your ego is entrenched in your work, you have perfectionistic and unrealistic standards that can stress you out. You might worry about aspects over which you have no control, like whether you will get promoted. By going beyond the self, you focus on overcoming challenges and delivering high-quality work.

TABLE C.1 Putting It All Together

Now that you've been exposed to the seven-step burnout solution, it's time to see how these steps can be applied together to your situation.

1. Emotional intelligence

Identify your unmet needs.

_____

Choose a self-affirming statement.

_____

How can you focus more on your strengths?

_____

What will you do to control your emotions more?

_____

2. Empowerment

What are the most important tasks to prioritize?

_____

What can you do to eliminate distractions?

_____

How can you harness more of what gives you power?

_____

How can you minimize energy drains?

_____

3. Engagement

How can you eliminate obstacles to optimal engagement?

_____

What can you do to attain more social support?

_____

How do you plan to increase personal resources (hope, efficacy, resilience, optimism)?

_____

What changes can you implement to better manage your time?

_____

4. Efficacy

Identify an area where you lack efficacy.

_____

What are some past accomplishments to consider?

_____

Given your past accomplishments, what encouraging statement can you make about yourself to build up your confidence in this identified area?

_____

What small action can you take to have a small win?

_____

5. Energy

☐ I take breaks throughout the day.
☐ I take vacations at least once per year where I unplug from work.
☐ I recognize that my productivity does not define my worth.
☐ I have healthy boundaries in place that ensure I incorporate self-care.

6. Effort

☐ My job provides me with inner rewards.
☐ I focus on what I want rather than what I don't want.
☐ I maintain a clutter-free work environment.
☐ I fill my mind with positive thoughts and gratitude.

7. Enlightenment

☐ I train my mind through regular meditation and mindfulness practices.
☐ I focus on overcoming challenges and delivering high-quality work.
☐ I practice compassion with myself and others.
☐ I keep bringing my focus back to the present.

Finally, when you bring your heart into everything you do, you are genuinely present, compassionate, and calm. As a result, you will more easily connect with others and draw people and success to you.

MAKING SENSE OF IT ALL

The information presented as solutions to burnout can also be organized and understood in terms of energy. There are energy centers in your body called "dantians," according to Taoist tradition, or "chakras," according to Hindu tradition (figure C.1). While there are seven main chakras along the spine, we will focus on the ones that align with the three dantians. These centers of energy correspond with the proposed solutions to burnout.

Corresponding with the three Dantians

FIGURE C.1   The Seven-Step Solution to Burnout and the Chakra System.

The lower dantian (navel chakra) is the center of personal power, which gives you access to your gut to make informed decisions.

We began this book by talking about empowerment, engagement, efficacy, energy, and effort. These are all practices that strengthen you at the core, by which they augment the fire in your belly so that you can achieve what you desire.

Enlightenment and its associated practices are affiliated with the upper dantian (third-eye chakra), the area between your eyebrows and slightly up. This chakra is your center of vision, perception, logic, and intuition. When this energy center is balanced you are more prone to see the truth and access your intuitive knowing. This too can help you make good decisions.

In between the navel and third eye chakras lies the middle dantian (heart chakra). This area in the center of your chest is the area of love and compassion, which helps you connect with others. It accesses the relationship competencies of EQ to help you understand other people and engage with them. The heart chakra is also where you can practice self-love and find balance between giving and receiving. It is where all healing takes place, and it bridges your physical and spiritual life.

By focusing on these three meaningful energy centers, grounding and strengthening your core while also engaging the power of your mind will help you feel centered. Through the navel, third eye, and heart chakras you develop power, wisdom, and balance, respectively. Balance lies in the heart. This is where you not only know and master yourself but love yourself and your life.

When you utilize the Burnout Solution, you become *extraordinary*.

Next Steps

Challenge Yourself

Take the 7-Day Burnout to Your Best Life Bootcamp: www
.7dayburnoutchallenge.com.

Free Bonuses

Access additional helpful videos and downloads for free by vis-
iting www.BurnoutToResilience.com.

Connect with Me

Follow me on LinkedIn. Go to www.linkedin.com/in/sharon
grossman and click FOLLOW.

Pay It Forward

Some of the most meaningful experiences of my life have been
unexpected outreaches from friends in time of need. Like when
my family had COVID, and our neighbor dropped off chicken
soup at our doorstep. Those little acts of kindness are seldom
forgotten.

There's something magical about helping others, but especially strangers. That's because without knowing whom you're
touching, you can appreciate the impact you have on another
life.

I've got just the thing to give you that magical experience,
an opportunity to help someone you've never met.

There's someone out there, similar to a past version of you:
struggling with stress, seeking balance, looking for ways to com-
bat burnout, but lost on where to begin. This is where you can
help.

My goal is to guide professionals and businesses on how to
thrive without burnout, but to do that, I need visibility. Book
covers and reviews are often the deciders. If you've appreciated

this book, please take a moment right now to leave a quick, honest review. It's free and takes less than a minute.

Your review can aid in:

- Making one more life stress-free and fulfilled
- Helping an exhausted employee regain their energy
- Assisting a company in reducing turnover and increasing productivity

All it takes is a minute to leave a review, wherever you purchased your copy of this book.

Dr. Sharon Grossman

Acknowledgments

It would be foolish to attribute the winnings of any trophy to only the athlete. It is their coach, parent, team, and role models that help shape their success. Similarly, I have the honor and privilege to acknowledge those who helped shape this book into what it is today.

I would be remiss if I did not first name my husband, Marc—not because of his relationship to me, but because of his deep selflessness and understanding. Without missing a beat, anytime I explained that I needed to write, he would find ways to make it possible. He never questioned me or complained about my expressed needs. His unwavering support truly touches my heart.

I have been tremendously lucky to have my loving and supportive parents, Edna and Jerry. They have been by my side throughout the writing of this book, supporting me even though they knew nothing of the book's contents. Thank you, dearly.

I have learned so much from the challenges faced by my clients, who were brave enough to share their journeys with me and entrusted me with coaching them through the tough times. Your stories are what, I believe, will help readers of this book better understand the concepts outlined. I thank you for allowing me to share them.

Every good coach needs a coach, and I have been so fortunate to work with and be inspired by Maryann Ehman and Michelle Kulp, whose guidance and wisdom have lightened my load through the writing and publishing of this book.

I am also indebted to all the support staff who helped take this manuscript and liven it up, including my editors, Nicole Cosgrove and Karin Conn, and my designers, Gaudencio Canta,

Una Salimovic, and Badsha Bulbul. I am grateful for your patience, talent, and creativity.

This book would not be as comprehensive a workbook as it is without the helpful recommendations of my friend Surya. Thank you for taking the time to read my manuscript and provide me with detailed suggestions on how to improve it. Your advice to "make the reader work" resonated strongly.

Throughout these chapters I have briefly mentioned Samvara's name. He is my spiritual teacher, and many of these teachings are credited to him. Thank you for your wisdom and for broadening my understanding of what truly matters.

Lastly, I want to acknowledge you, the reader. It takes courage to admit you need help. Thank you for taking the time to read this. I hope this book helps you out of burnout and leads you to live life the way it was meant to be lived.

Notes

1. The Stress-Burnout Continuum

Epigraph: Richard S. Lazarus, *Psychological Stress and the Coping Process* (New York: McGraw-Hill, 1966).

1. Peter G. Nixon, "The Human Function Curve. With Special Reference to Cardiovascular Disorders: Part 1," *Practitioner* 217, no. 1301 (1976): 765–770.

2. Suzanne C. Kobassa, Salvatore R. Maddi, and Sheila Courington, "Personality and Constitution as Mediators in the Stress-Illness Relationship," *Journal of Health and Social Behaviour* 22, no. 4 (1981): 368–378.

2. Identifying Burnout Triggers

1. Evangelia Demerouti, Arnold B. Bakker, Friedhelm Nachreiner, and Wilmar B. Schaufeli, "The Job Demands–Resources Model of Burnout," *Journal of Applied Psychology* 86, no. 3 (2001): 499–512.

2. Lydia Saad, "The '40-Hour' Workweek Is Actually Longer—by Seven Hours," Gallup, August 29, 2014, https://news.gallup.com/poll/175286/hour-workweek-actually-longer-seven-hours.aspx.

3. "Average Working Week U.S. by Industry 2024," Statista, October 2024, www.statista.com/statistics/261808/monthly-change-of-the-average-working-week-of-all-us-employees-by-industry/.

4. "10 Statistics on Work-Life Balance That May Surprise You (2024)," Apollo Technical, 2024, www.apollotechnical.com/statistics-on-work-life-balance/.

5. John Pencavel, "The Productivity of Working Hours," IZA Discussion Paper Series no. 8129 (2014), https://docs.iza.org/dp8129.pdf.

6. Jena McGregor, "Feel Pressure to Work after Hours? You May Be Less Productive, Not More," *Forbes*, December 5, 2023, www.forbes.com/sites/jenamcgregor/2023/12/05/feel-pressure-to-work-after-hours-you-may-be-less-productive-not-more/.

7. Demerouti et al., "The Job Demands–Resources Model of Burnout."

8. Miron Zuckerman, Joseph Porac, Drew Lathin, and Edward L. Deci, "On the Importance of Self-Determination for Intrinsically Motivated Behaviour," *Personality and Social Psychology Bulletin* 4, no. 3 (1978): 443–446.

9. Arnold B. Bakker and Evangelia Demerouti, "The Job Demands–Resources Model: State of the Art," *Journal of Managerial Psychology* 22, no. 3 (2007): 309–328.

10. Marcie A. Cavanaugh, Wendy R. Boswell, Mark V. Roehling, and John W. Boudreau, "An Empirical Examination of Self-Reported Work Stress among U.S. Managers," *Journal of Applied Psychology* 85, no. 1 (2000): 65–74.

11. Haim H. Gaziel, "Determinants of Perceived Deficiency of Autonomy among Elementary School Administrators," *Social Behavior and Personality: An International Journal* 17, no. 1 (1989): 57–66.

12. Edward L. Deci and Richard M. Ryan, "The Support of Autonomy and the Control of Behaviour," *Journal of Personality and Social Psychology* 53, no. 6 (1988): 1024.

13. Robert A. Karasek, "Job Demands, Job Decision Latitude, and Mental Strain: Implications for Job Redesign," *Administrative Science Quarterly* 24, no. 2 (1979): 285.

14. Dragan Mijakoski, Jovanka Karadzhinska-Bislimovska, Sasho Stoleski, Jordan Minov, Aneta Atanasovska, and Elida Bihorac, "Job Demands, Burnout, and Teamwork in Healthcare Professionals Working in a General Hospital That Was Analysed at Two Points in Time," *Open Access Macedonian Journal of Medical Sciences* 6, no. 4 (2018): 723–729.

15. Richard S. Lazarus and Susan Folkman, *Stress, Appraisal, and Coping* (New York: Springer, 1984).

16. Christina Maslach and Michael P. Leiter, *The Truth about Burnout: How Organizations Cause Personal Stress and What to Do about It* (San Francisco: Jossey-Bass, 1997).

17. Robert L. Kahn, *Organizational Stress: Studies in Role Conflict and Ambiguity* (Oxford: John Wiley, 1964).

18. Adeboye T. Ayinde and Aderami Obawole, "Pay Satisfaction and Role Ambiguity as Predictors of Burnout among Osun State Civil Servants, Nigeria," *European Scientific Journal* 15, no. 8 (2019): 1018–1027.

19. Lazarus and Folkman, Stress, *Appraisal and Coping*.

3. Recognizing Burnout Signs

1. Steven Stack, "Suicide Risk among Physicians: A Multivariate Analysis," *Archives of Suicide Research* 8, no. 3 (2004): 287–292.

2. Brené Brown, *Rising Strong: How the Ability to Reset Transforms the Way We Live, Love, Parent, and Lead* (New York: Random House, 2017).

3. Marc Van Veldoven and Sjaak Broersen, "Measurement Quality and Validity of the 'Need for Recovery Scale,'" *Occupational and Environmental Medicine* 60, no. 1 (2003): i3–i9.

4. Robert A. Karasek, "Job Demands," *Administrative Science Quarterly* 24, no. 2 (1979): 285; Herbert J. Freudenberger and Gail North, *Women's*

Burnout: How to Spot It, How to Reverse It, and How to Prevent It (Garden City, NY: Doubleday, 1985), in Ulrich Kraft, "Burned Out," *Scientific American Mind* 17, no. 3 (2006): 28–33.

4. Self-Awareness

1. Myers & Briggs Company, "Myers-Briggs Type Indicator (MBTI)," accessed September 19, 2019, https://www.themyersbriggs.com/en-US/Products-and-Services/Myers-Briggs.

2. Abraham H. Maslow, "A Theory of Human Motivation." *Psychological Review* 50, no. 4 (1943): 370–396.

3. R. Douglas Fields, *Why We Snap: Understanding the Rage Circuit in Your Brain* (New York: Baker & Taylor, 2016).

4. "List of Maladaptive Schemas," Wikipedia, accessed September 19, 2019, https://en.m.wikipedia.org/wiki/List_of_maladaptive_schemas.

5. Emotional Literacy

1. Daniel J. Siegel, *Mindsight: The New Science of Personal Transformation* (New York: Bantam Books, 2010).

6. Emotional Mastery

1. Malcolm Gladwell, *Outliers: A Story of Success* (New York: Back Bay Books, 2011).

2. Corrie Ten Boom with Jamie Buckingham, *Tramp for the Lord* (London: Hodder and Stoughton, 1975).

3. Brené Brown, *The Call to Courage*, directed by Sandra Restrepo, streaming video (Netflix, 2019).

4. A. Creed Torrey, Jarrod Reisweber, and Aaron T. Beck, *Cognitive Therapy for Adolescents in School Settings* (New York: Guilford, 2011).

5. Ilona Jerabek, "Self-Controlled vs. Emotionally Constipated: Study Reveals the Drawbacks of a Lack of Emotional Experience," PR Web, June 23, 2018, https://www.prweb.com/releases/2018/06/prweb15583282.htm.

7. Zone of Optimal Performance

1. As discussed in Eric Barker, *Barking up the Wrong Tree: The Surprising Science behind Why Everything You Know about Success Is (Mostly) Wrong* (New York: HarperOne, 2017).

8. Empathy

1. Sergei Prokofiev, *Peter and the Wolf* (New York: Random House, 2004).

2. Quoted in Daniel H. Pink, *Drive: The Surprising Truth about What Motivates Us* (Edinburgh: Canongate Books, 2018), 143.

3. Emma Seppälä and Marissa King, "Burnout at Work Isn't Just about Exhaustion. It's Also about Loneliness," *Harvard Business Review*, June 29, 2017.

4. Caren Baruch-Feldman, Elizabeth Brondolo, Dena Ben-Dayan, and Joseph Schwartz, "Sources of Social Support and Burnout, Job Satisfaction, and Productivity," *Journal of Occupational Health Psychology* 7, no. 1 (2002): 84–93.

5. "12 Ways Nurses Can Beat Compassion Fatigue," *Nurse Buff* (blog), September 12, 2015, https://online.hpu.edu/blog/burnout-vs-compassion-fatigue.

9. Relationship Management

1. Marsha M. Linehan, *DBT Skills Training Manual* (New York: Guilford, 2017).

2. Robert B. Cialdini, *Influence: The Psychology of Persuasion* (New York: Collins, 2007).

10. The Essentials of Effective Communication

1. William R. Miller and Stephen Rollnick, *Motivational Interviewing: Preparing People for Change* (New York: Guilford, 2002).

2. William R. Miller, Cheryl A. Taylor, and JoAnne C. West, "Focused versus Broad-Spectrum Behavior Therapy for Problem Drinkers," *Journal of Consulting and Clinical Psychology* 48, no. 5 (1980): 590–601.

3. The Dalai Lama and Paul Ekman, *Emotional Awareness: Overcoming the Obstacles to Psychological Balance and Compassion; A Conversation between the Dalai Lama and Paul Ekman* (New York: Times Books, 2008).

Step 2. Empowerment

Epigraph: Jim Loehr and Tony Schwartz, *The Power of Full Engagement: Managing Energy, Not Time, Is the Key to High Performance and Personal Renewal* (New York: Free Press, 2003).

11. Personal Power

1. Justin Yang, Costas A. Christophi, Andrea Farioli, Dorothee M. Baur, et al., "Association between Push-Up Exercise Capacity and Future Cardiovascular Events among Active Adult Men," *JAMA Network Open* 2, no. 2 (2019): e190035, https://jamanetwork.com/journals/jamanetworkopen/fullarticle/2724778.

2. Quoted in Andrew Unterberger, "10 Reasons Peter Gabriel's 'Solsbury Hill' Is One of the Greatest Songs of All Time," *Billboard*, February 25, 2017, https://www.billboard.com/articles/columns/rock/7702117/peter-gabriel-solsbury-hill-anniversary-greatest-song.

12. Amplifying Your Personal Power

1. Alethia Luna, "6 Types of Energy Vampires That Emotionally Exhaust You," *LonerWolf*, December 13, 2019, https://lonerwolf.com/types-energy-vampire/.

13. Becoming More Yourself

1. Murray Bowen, *Family Therapy in Clinical Practice* (New York: Jason Aronson, 1978).

14. Hierarchy of Needs

1. Abraham H. Maslow, "A Theory of Human Motivation," *Psychological Review* 50, no. 4 (1943): 370–396.

2. Bronnie Ware, *The Top Five Regrets of the Dying: A Life Transformed by the Dearly Departing* (Carlsbad, CA: Hay House Australia, 2019).

3. Candace B. Pert, *Molecules of Emotion* (New York: Scribner, 1997).

4. Quoted in Volney Streamer, *In Friendship's Name* (New York: Brentanos, 1909), 22.

5. Tom Rath, *Vital Friends: The People You Can't Afford to Live Without* (New York: Gallup Press, 2006).

6. Mel Robbins, *Stop Saying You're Fine: The No-BS Guide to Getting What You Want* (New York: Three Rivers Press, 2006).

15. Poor Engagement

1. Christina Maslach, "Burned-Out," *Human Behavior* 5, no. 9 (1976): 16–22.

2. Gallup, "State of the American Workplace," 2018, news.gallup.com/reports/199961/state-american-workplace-report-2017.aspx.

3. Employer Flexible, "COVID-19 Crisis Spurs U.S. Employee Engagement to Record Highs," 2020, www.employerflexible.com/insights/covid-19-crisis-spurs-u-s-employee-engagement-to-record-highs/.

4. Gallup, "U.S. Employee Engagement Rises Slightly in Q2 2024," 2024, www.gallup.com/workplace/350157/employee-engagement-rise-q2-2024.aspx.

16. Three Dimensions of Optimal Engagement

1. Wilmar B. Schaufeli, Marisa Salanova, and Vincente Gonzáles-Romá, "The Measurement of Engagement and Burnout: A Two Sample Confirmatory Factor Analytic Approach," *Journal of Happiness Studies* 3, no. 1 (2002): 71–92, https://link.springer.com/article/10.1023/A:1015630930326.

2. Jari J. Hakanen, Maria C. W. Peters, and Wilmar B. Schaufeli, "Different Types of Employee Well-Being across Time and Their Relationships with Job Crafting," *Journal of Occupational Health Psychology* 23, no. 2 (2018): 289–301, https://www.ncbi.nlm.nih.gov/pubmed/28191997.

3. Mihaly Csikszentmihalyi, *Flow: The Psychology of Optimal Experience* (New York: Harper and Row, 2009).

17. Being In the Flow

Epigraph: Mihaly Csikszentmihalyi, *Flow: The Psychology of Optimal Experience* (New York: Harper and Row, 2009).

1. Csikszentmihalyi, *Flow*.

2. Csikszentmihalyi, *Flow*.

3. Lao Tzu, *Tao Te Ching*, trans. Stephen Mitchell (New York: Harmony Books, 1988).

4. Mihaly Csikszentmihalyi, *Flow and the Foundations of Positive Psychology: The Collected Works of Mihaly Csikszentmihalyi* (Dordrecht: Springer, 2016), 145.

18. Maximizing Job Resources

1. Wilmar B. Schaufeli, "Applying the Job Demands–Resources Model: A 'How To' Guide to Measuring and Tackling Work Engagement and Burnout," *Organizational Dynamics* 46 (2017): 121, https://www.wilmarschaufeli.nl/publications/Schaufeli/476.pdf.

2. Schaufeli, "Applying the Job Demands–Resources Model," 123.

3. Jerzy Koniarek and Bohdan Dudek, "Social Support as a Buffer in the Stress–Burnout Relationship," *International Journal of Stress Management* 3, no. 2 (1996): 99–106, https://link.springer.com/article/10.1007/BF01857718.

4. Lebena S. Varghese, Arielle P. Rogers, Lisa Finkelstein, and Larissa K. Barber, "Examining Mentors as Buffers of Burnout for Employees High in Neuroticism," *Human Resource Development Quarterly* 31, no. 3 (2020): 281–288.

5. Lillian T. Eby, Marcus Butts, and Angie Lockwood, "Predictors of Success in the Era of the Boundaryless Career," *Journal of Organizational Behavior* 24, no. 6 (2003): 689–708.

6. Christine Porath, "Why Being Respectful to Your Coworkers Is Good for Business," TED Talk, January 2018, https://www.ted.com/talks /christine_porath_why_being_respectful_to_your_coworkers_is_good _for_business?subtitle=en.

7. Porath, "Why Being Respectful to Your Coworkers Is Good for Business."

8. Lexy Adkins, "How Do Employees Assess Fairness?," DeGarmo Group, November 8, 2019, https://www.degarmo.com/how-do-employees -assess-fairness.

9. Jim Collins, *Good to Great* (London: Random House Business, 2001).

19. Leveraging Personal Resources

1. Fred Luthans, Kyle W. Luthans, and Brett C. Luthans, "Positive Psychological Capital: Beyond Human and Social Capital," *Business Horizons* 47, no. 1 (2004): 45–50, https://doi.org/10.1016/j.bushor.2003.11.007.

2. C. R. Snyder et al., "The Will and the Ways: Development and Validation of an Individual-Differences Measure of Hope," *Journal of Personality and Social Psychology* 60, no. 4 (1991): 570–585, https://ou.edu/content /dam/Tulsa/research/The-Will-and-the-Ways_Validation-of-Hope_Snyder .pdf.

3. Leland Beaumont, "Hope," Emotional Competency, 2005–2009, http:// www.emotionalcompetency.com/hope.htm.

4. Jim C. Collins, *Good to Great* (London: Random House Business, 2001), 83–87.

5. Fred Luthans, Carolyn M. Youssef-Morgan, and Bruce J. Avolio, *Psychological Capital and Beyond* (Oxford: Oxford University Press, 2015).

6. Albert Bandura, "Self-Efficacy Mechanism in Human Agency," *American Psychologist* 37, no. 2 (1982): 122–147, https://psycnet.apa.org/record /1982-25814-001.

7. Charles Darwin with David Quammen, *On the Origin of Species* (New York: Sterling Signature, 2011).

8. Carole Dweck, *Mindset* (London: Robinson, 2017).

9. Victor E. Frankl, *Man's Search for Meaning: An Introduction to Logotherapy* (London: Hodder and Stoughton, 1962).

10. John Boyd and Philip Zimbardo, *The Time Paradox: The New Psychology of Time That Will Change Your Life* (London: Rider, 2009).

11. Nan Henderson and Mike M. Milstein, *Resiliency in Schools: Making It Happen for Students and Educators* (Thousand Oaks, CA: Corwin Press, 2003).

12. K. M. Connor and J. R. T. Davidson, "Development of a New Resilience Scale: The Connor-Davidson Resilience Scale," *Depression and Anxiety* 18, no. 2 (2003): 76–82, https://doi.org/10.1002/da.10113.

13. Janet Stevens and Aesop, *The Tortoise and the Hare: An Aesop Fable* (New York Holiday House, 1984).

14. Brené Brown, *The Gifts of Imperfection: Let Go of Who You Think You're Supposed to Be and Embrace Who You Are* (Center City, MN: Hazelden, 2010).

15. Lise Solberg Nes and S. C. Segerstrom, "Dispositional Optimism and Coping: A Meta-Analytic Review," *Personality and Social Psychology Review* 10, no. 3 (2006): 235–251, https://doi.org/10.1207/s15327957pspr1003_3.

16. Glenn Affleck, Howard Tennen, and Andrea Apter, "Optimism, Pessimism, and Daily Life with Chronic Illness," in *Optimism & Pessimism: Implications for Theory, Research, and Practice*, ed. E. C. Chang (Washington, DC: American Psychological Association, 2001), 147–168.

17. Gabriele Prati and Luca Pietrantoni, "Optimism, Social Support, and Coping Strategies as Factors Contributing to Posttraumatic Growth," *Journal of Loss and Trauma* 14, no. 5 (2009): 364–388, https://doi.org/10.1080/15325020902724271.

18. Nathan M. Radcliffe and William M. P. Klein, "Dispositional, Unrealistic, and Comparative Optimism: Differential Relations with the Knowledge and Processing of Risk Information and Beliefs about Personal Risk," *Personality and Social Psychology Bulletin* 28, no. 6 (2002): 836–846, https://doi.org/10.1177/0146167202289012.

19. Leslie P. Kamen and Martin E. P. Seligman, "Explanatory Style and Health," *Current Psychology* 6, no. 3 (1987): 207–218, https://doi.org/10.1007/BF02686648.

20. Richard E. Lucas, Ed Diener, and Eunkook Suh, "Discriminant Validity of Well-Being Measures," *Journal of Personality and Social Psychology* 71, no. 3 (1996): 616–628, https://doi.org/10.1037/0022-3514.71.3.616.

21. Michael E. McCullough, Robert A. Emmons, and JoAnn Tsang, "The Grateful Disposition: A Conceptual and Empirical Topography," *Journal of Personality and Social Psychology* 82, no. 1 (2002): 112–127, https://doi.org/10.1037//0022- 3514.82.1.112; Sara B. Algoe and Jonathan Haidt, "Witnessing Excellence in Action: The 'Other- Praising' Emotions of Elevation, Gratitude, and Admiration," *Journal of Positive Psychology* 4, no. 2 (2009): 105–127, https://doi.org/10.1080/17439760802650519.

22. Yik-man Wong, Jesse Owen, Nicole T. Gabana, et al., "Does Gratitude Writing Improve the Mental Health of Psychotherapy Clients? Evidence from a Randomized Controlled Trial," *Psychotherapy Research* 28, no. 2 (March 2016): 192–202, https://doi.org/10.1080/10503307.2016.1169332.

23. Lung Hung Chen and Chiahuei Wu, "Gratitude Enhances Change in Athletes' Self-Esteem: The Moderating Role of Trust in Coach," *Journal of Applied Sport Psychology* 26, no. 3 (2014): 349–362, https://doi.org/10.1080/10413200.2014.889255.

24. Patrick L. Hill, Mathias Allemand, and Brent W. Roberts, "Examining the Pathways between Gratitude and Self-Rated Physical Health across Adulthood," *Personality and Individual Differences* 54, no. 1 (2013): 92–96, https://doi.org/10.1016/j.paid.2012.08.011.

25. Alex M. Wood, Stephen Joseph, Joanna Lloyd, and Samuel Adkins, "Gratitude Influences Sleep through the Mechanism of Pre-Sleep Cognitions," *Journal of Psychosomatic Research* 66, no. 1 (2009): 43–48, https://doi.org/10.1016/j.jpsychores.2008.09.002.

26. Philip C. Watkins, Kathrane Woodward, Tamara Stone, and Russell L. Kolts, "Gratitude and Happiness: Development of a Measure of Gratitude, and Relationship with Subjective Well-Being," *Social Behaviorand Personality: An International Journal* 31, no. 5 (2003): 431–452, https://doi.org/10.2224/sbp.2003.31.5.431.

27. Nathan DeWall, Nathaniel M. Lambert, Richard S. Pond Jr., Todd B. Kashdan, and Frank D. Fincham, "A Grateful Heart Is a Nonviolent Heart," *Social Psychological and Personality Science* 3, no. 2 (2011): 232–240, https://doi.org/10.1177/1948550611416675.

28. Sara B. Algoe, B. L. Fredrickson, and S. L. Gable, "The Social Functions of the Emotion of Gratitude via Expression," *Emotion* 13, no. 4 (2013): 605–609, https://psycnet.apa.org/record/2008-07784-028.

29. Algoe, Fredrickson, and Gable, "The Social Functions of Gratitude."

30. Sara B. Algoe, "Find, Remind, and Bind: The Functions of Gratitude in Everyday Relationships," *Social and Personality Psychology Compass* 6, no. 6 (2012): 455–469, https://doi.org/10.1111/j.1751-9004.2012.00439.x.

31. Michael Craig Miller, "In Praise of Gratitude," *Harvard Health Blog*, November 21, 2012, https://www.health.harvard.edu/mind-and-mood/in-praise-of-gratitude.

20. Mastering Time Management

1. Stephen R. Covey, *The 7 Habits of Highly Effective People: Restoring the Character Ethic* (New York: Simon and Schuster, 1989).

2. Eric Carle, *The Very Busy Spider* (New York: Philomel Books, 1984).

3. "What Is Pomodoro Technique Time Management?," TechTarget, https://www.techtarget.com/whatis/definition/pomodoro-technique, accessed November 7, 2024.

4. Rescuetime tool, http://rescuetime.com, accessed March 16, 2019.

5. Michael J. A. Wohl, Timothy A. Pychyl, and Shannon H. Bennett, "I Forgive Myself, Now I Can Study: How Self-Forgiveness for Procrastinating Can Reduce Future Procrastination," *Personality and Individual Differences* 48, no. 7 (2010): 803–808, https://doi.org/10.1016/j.paid.2010.01.029.

Step 4. Efficacy

1. Albert Bandura, *Self-Efficacy: The Exercise of Control* (New York: W. H. Freeman, 1997).

21. Self-Efficacy Spirals

1. Michael Masuch, "Vicious Circles in Organizations," *Administrative Science Quarterly* 30, no. 3 (1985): 14–23, https://www.jstor.org/stable/2392809?seq=1.

22. How Spirals Get Started

1. Dana H. Lindsley, Daniel J. Brass, and James B. Thomas, "Efficacy-Performance Spirals: A Multilevel Perspective," *Academy of Management Review* 20, no. 3 (1995): 650, https://doi.org/10.2307/258790.

23. What Keeps Spirals Going

1. Dana H. Lindsley, Daniel J. Brass, and James B. Thomas, "Efficacy-Performance Spirals: A Multilevel Perspective," *Academy of Management Review* 20, no. 3 (1995): 645–678, https://doi.org/10.2307/258790.

2. Quoted in J. L. Elkhorne, "Edison—The Fabulous Drone," *73 Magazine* 46, no. 3 (March 1967): 52–54, http://www.arimi.it/wp-content/73/03_March_1967.pdf.

3. Robert Rosenthal and Lenore Jacobson, "Pygmalion in the Classroom," *The Urban Review* 3, no. 1 (1968): 16–20, https://link.springer.com/article/10.1007/BF02322211.

24. How to Stop a Downward Spiral

1. Dana H. Lindsley, Daniel J. Brass, and James B. Thomas. "Efficacy-Performance Spirals: A Multilevel Perspective," *Academy of Management Review* 20, no. 3 (1995): 662, https://doi.org/10.2307/258790.

2. Teresa M. Amabile and Steven J. Kramer, *The Progress Principle: Using Small Wins to Ignite Joy, Engagement, and Creativity at Work* (Boston: Harvard Business Review Press, 2011).

25. Mindset Obstacles to Self-Care

1. Matthew Thorpe and Rachael Ajmera, "How Meditation Benefits Your Mind and Body," *Healthline*, August 15, 2024, https://www.healthline.com/nutrition/12-benefits-of-meditation.

26. Managing Your Energy

1. J. M. Ellenbogen, J. D. Payne, and R. Stickgold, "The Role of Sleep in Declarative Memory Consolidation: Passive, Permissive, Active or None?," *Current Opinion in Neurobiology* 16, no. 6 (2006): 716–722, https://doi.org/10.1016/j.conb.2006.10.006.

2. "Benefits of Moderate Sun Exposure," Harvard Health Publishing. January 20, 2017, https://www.health.harvard.edu/diseases-and-conditions/benefits-of-moderate-sun-exposure.

3. Michael A. Smith, Alexandra Thompson, Lynsey J. Hall, Sarah F. Allen, and Mark A. Wetherell, "The Physical and Psychological Health Benefits of Positive Emotional Writing: Investigating the Moderating Role of Type D (Distressed) Personality," *British Journal of Health Psychology* 23, no. 4 (2018): 857–871.

4. S. Leikas and V. J. Ilmarinen, "Happy Now, Tired Later? Extraverted and Conscientious Behavior Are Related to Immediate Mood Gains, But to Later Fatigue," *Journal of Personality* 85, no. 5 (2016): 603–615, https://doi.org/ 10.1111/jopy.12264.

27. Establishing Healthy Boundaries

Epigraph: Oprah Winfrey, *The Wisdom of Sundays: Life-Changing Insights from Super Soul Conversations* (New York: Flatiron Books, 2017).

1. Shel Silverstein, *The Giving Tree* (New York: HarperCollins, 1992), 27.

2. "Dr. David Gruder Nonprofit Exchange," YouTube, February 27, 2017, https://www.youtube.com/watch?list=PLruEzkHGNTZ4bt2XgrpQFR6_GGrBKpsGm&time_continue=1184&v=1u3ls59du58.

3. See discussion in R. Skip Johnson, "Escaping Conflict and the Drama Triangle," BDP Family, January 4, 2018, https://www.bpdfamily.com/content /karpman-drama-triangle.

28. Transitioning Out of Work Mode

1. U.S. Travel Association, "Paid Time-Off Trends in the U.S.," fact sheet, 2018, https://www.ustravel.org/sites/default/files/media_root/document /Paid%20Time%20Off%20Trends%20Fact%20Sheet.pdf.

2. U.S. Office of Personnel Management, "In Lieu of Holidays for Employees on Alternative Work Schedules," www.opm.gov/policy-data-oversight /pay-leave/work-schedules/fact-sheets/Federal-Holidays-In-Lieu-Of-De termination, accessed November 11, 2024.

3. U.S. Travel Association, "Paid Time-Off Trends in the U.S."

Step 6. Effort

Epigraph: Jason Fried and David Heinemeier Hansson, *Rework* (New York: Crown Business, 2010).

29. Smart Effort

1. Theodore Melfi, dir., *Hidden Figures* (20th Century Fox, 2016).

2. Greg Smith, "Why I Am Leaving Goldman Sachs," *New York Times*, March 14, 2012, https://www.nytimes.com/2012/03/14/opinion/why-i-am -leaving-goldman-sachs.html.

3. Christina Maslach, "Burned-Out," *Human Relations* 9, no. 5 (1976): 16–22.

4. Hely Innanen, Asko Tolvanen, and Katariina Salmela-Aro, "Burnout, Work Engagement and Workaholism among Highly Educated Employees: Profiles, Antecedents and Outcomes," *Burnout Research* 1, no. 1 (2014): 38– 49, https://doi.org/10.1016/j.burn.2014.04.001.

5. Leon Festinger and James M. Carlsmith, "Cognitive Consequences of Forced Compliance," *Journal of Abnormal and Social Psychology* 58, no. 2 (1959): 203–210, https://faculty.washington.edu/jdb/345/345%20Articles /Festinger%20&%20Carlsmith.pdf.

6. Natasja Van Vegchel, Jan de Jong, and Paul A. Landsbergis, "Occupational Stress in (Inter)action: The Interplay between Job Demands and Job Resources," *Journal of Organizational Behaviour* 26, no. 5 (2005): 535–560, https://doi.org/ 10.1002/job.327.

7. Christina Maslach and Michael P. Leiter, *The Truth about Burnout: How Organizations cause Personal Stress and What to Do about It* (San Francisco: Jossey-Bass, 2000).

8. Esther Hicks and Jerry Hicks, *Ask and It Is Given: Learning to Manifest Your Desires* (Carlsbad, CA: Hay House, 2004).

30. Right Effort

1. *Merriam-Webster's Dictionary*, "Eightfold Path," https://www.merriam -webster.com/dictionary/Eightfold%20Path, accessed August 28, 2019.

2. Mark Nathaniel Bing, "The Integrative Model of Personality Assessment for Achievement Motivation and Fear of Failure: Implications for the Prediction of Effort and Performance" (PhD diss., University of Tennessee, 2002), http://trace.tennessee.edu/cgi/viewcontent.cgi?article=3536&context =utk_graddiss.

3. BBC, "Buddhism at a Glance," November 17, 2009, https://www.bbc .co.uk/religion/religions/buddhism/ataglance/glance.shtm.

4. Samvara, "How to Do Buddhism, Satsang with Samvara" (lecture, Fort Mason Center, San Francisco, CA, October 27, 2018).

5. Samvara, "How to Do Buddhism."

6. Samvara, "How to Do Buddhism."

7. Daniel Goleman and Richard J. Davidson, *Altered Traits: Science Reveals How Meditation Changes Your Mind, Brain, and Body* (New York: Avery, 2017), 17.

8. Daniel Duane, "El Capitan, My El Capitan," *New York Times*, June 9, 2017, https://www.nytimes.com/2017/06/09/opinion/el-capitan-my-el-capitan .html.

9. Samvara, "How to Do Buddhism."

Step 7. Enlightenment

Epigraph: Rumi, *The Essential Rumi*, trans. Coleman Barks (San Francisco: Harper, 1995).

31. What Is Enlightenment?

1. Aaron Antonovsky, *Health, Stress, and Coping* (San Francisco: Jossey-Bass, 1980).

32. Why Enlightenment Is Important

1. Abraham Maslow, "A Theory of Human Motivation," *Psychological Review* 50, no. 4 (1943): 370–396.

2. Scott R. Baker et al., "The Power of Proximity to Coworkers: Training for Tomorrow or Productivity Today?" (National Bureau of Economic

Research Working Paper no. 31880, February 2023), https://www.nber .org/papers/w31880.

3. Eric Barker, *Barking Up the Wrong Tree: The Surprising Science behind Why Everything You Know about Success Is (Mostly) Wrong* (New York: Harper-One, 2017).

33. Living on Purpose

Epigraph: Pico Iyer, *The Art of Stillness: Adventures in Going Nowhere* (New York: Simon and Schuster, 2014).

1. Huan Song et al., "Association of Stress-Related Disorders with Subsequent Autoimmune Disease," *JAMA* 319, no. 23 (2018): 2388–2400, https://jamanetwork.com/journals/jama/fullarticle/2685155.

2. Mika Kivimäki et al., "Work Stress and Risk of Death in Men and Women with and without Cardiometabolic Disease: A Multicohort Study," *The Lancet Diabetes & Endocrinology* 6, no. 9 (2018): 705–713, https://www .thelancet.com/pdfs/journals/landia/PIIS2213-8587(18)30140-2.pdf.

34. How You Can Reach Enlightenment

Epigraph: Pico Iyer, *The Art of Stillness: Adventures in Going Nowhere* (New York: Simon and Schuster, 2014).

1. Seth Godin, "On Feeling Like a Failure," *Seth's Blog*, October 15, 2015, https://seths.blog/2015/10/on-feeling-like-a-failure/.

35. Integrating Enlightenment Practices

Epigraph: Joseph Brodsky, *Less Than One: Selected Essays* (New York: Farrar, Straus, Giroux, 1986).

1. Justin M. Berg, Jane E. Dutton, and Amy Wrzesniewski, "What Is Job Crafting and Why Does It Matter?" (Ann Arbor: Positive Organizational Scholarship, University of Michigan, August 1, 2008), https://positiveorgs .bus.umich.edu/wp-content/uploads/What-is-Job-Crafting-and-Why-Does -it-Matter1.pdf.

2. Gordon L. Flett, Paul H. Hewitt, Brenley Shapiro, and Jill Rayman, "Perfectionism, Beliefs, and Adjustment in Dating Relationships," *Current Psychology* 20, no. 4 (2001): 289–311, https://link.springer.com/article/10.1007 /s12144-001-1013-4.

3. Seth Godin, "The Illusion of Control." *Seth's Blog*, August 5, 2015, https://seths.blog/2015/08/the-illusion-of-control/.

4. Barry Schwartz, *Why We Work* (London: Simon and Schuster, 2015), 1–2.

5. David Gelles, *Mindful Work: How Meditation Is Changing Business from the Inside Out* (Boston: Eamon Dolon and Houghton Mifflin Harcourt, 2015).

6. Laura Shin, "Secret Way to Boost the Corporate Bottom Line," *The Fiscal Times*, September 25, 2012, http://www.thefiscaltimes.com/Articles /2012/09/25/Secret-Way-to-Boost-the-Corporate-Bottom-Line.

7. John Hilton, "Why Mindfulness Works Wonders," *Australasian Lawyer*, February 17, 2016, https://www.thelawyermag.com/au/news/general /why-mindfulness-works-wonders/199457.

8. Daniel Goleman and Richard J. Davidson, *Altered Traits: Science Reveals How Meditation Changes Your Mind, Brain, and Body* (New York: Avery, 2017).

9. Jo Cutler and Daniel Campbell-Meiklejohn, "A Comparative fMRI Meta-Analysis of Altruistic and Strategic Decision to Give," *NeuroImage* 184, no. 1 (2019): 227–241, https://www.ncbi.nlm.nih.gov/pubmed/30195947.

10. Cutler and Campbell-Meiklejohn, "A Comparative fMRI Meta-Analysis."

11. Hamdi Ulukaya, "The Anti-CEO Playbook," TED: Ideas Worth Spreading, April 2019, https://www.ted.com/talks/hamdi_ulukaya_the_an ti_ceo_playbook?language=en.

12. "Death of a Genius: His Fourth Dimension, Time, Overtakes Einstein," in *Old Man's Advice to Youth: "Never Lose a Holy Curiosity,"* ed. William Miller (New York: Time, 1955), 64.

Exercise for Step 7

1. Daniel Goleman and Richard J. Davidson, *Altered Traits: Science Reveals How Meditation Changes Your Mind, Brain, and Body* (New York: Avery, 2017).

Conclusion

Epigraph: Portia Nelson, *There's a Hole in My Sidewalk: The Romance of Self-Discovery* (Hillsboro, OR: Beyond Words, 1993).

Index

Note: Page numbers in *italics* indicate figures and tables.

About the Author

Dr. Sharon Grossman is a psychologist, executive coach, keynote speaker, corporate trainer, business consultant, and burnout expert. After years of focusing on helping leaders recover from burnout, she's rededicated her career to helping organizations to create a thriving corporate culture so that their employees feel valued, engaged, and motivated to stay. That's because leadership plays a big role in both burnout and retention.

Known for her direct but compassionate and grounded nature, Dr. Sharon coaches her clients via video conferencing, online through her courses, and during specially designed workshops and retreats.

For more information and tools, visit www.drsharongrossman .com.